LIVING A REAL LIFE WITH REAL FOOD

LIVING A REAL LIFE WITH REAL FOOD

HOW TO GET HEALTHY, LOSE WEIGHT, AND STAY
ENERGIZED—THE KOSHER WAY

BETH WARREN, MS, RD, CDN

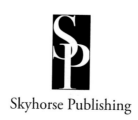

Skyhorse Publishing

Skyhorse Publishing books may be purchased in bulk at special discounts for sales promotion, corporate gifts, fund-raising, or educational purposes. Special editions can also be created to specifications. For details, contact the Special Sales Department, Skyhorse Publishing, 307 West 36th Street, 11th Floor, New York, NY 10018 or info@skyhorsepublishing.com.

Skyhorse® and Skyhorse Publishing® are registered trademarks of Skyhorse Publishing, Inc.®, a Delaware corporation.

www.skyhorsepublishing.com

10 9 8 7 6 5 4 3 2 1

Library of Congress Cataloging-in-Publication Data

Warren, Beth, 1984-

Living a real life with real food: how to get healthy, lose weight, and stay energized, the kosher way / Beth Warren, MS, RD, CDN.

    pages cm

Includes bibliographical references.

ISBN 978-1-62636-571-1 (alk. paper)

1. Natural foods—Therapeutic use. 2. Kosher food. 3. Reducing diets—Recipes. I. Title.

RM237.55.W37 2014

613.2'65—dc23

                    2013034823

Printed in China

CONTENTS

THE KOSHER REAL-FOOD DIET FOUNDATION

"It is a mitzvah (commandment) for one to conduct himself with good measure and good habits and to maintain his health in order to be healthy and strong for the service of the Creator, may He be exalted."

—*The Tur*
(a commentator during the thirteenth century in Spain and the son of the Rosh, on the eleventh chapter in the book, The Laws of the Daily Conduct)

CHAPTER 1

MY KOSHER SONG

WHY REAL FOOD?

• •

The real-food diet. It sounds simple enough. Eat real foods.

Unfortunately, life is complicated. The simplicity got pushed beneath all the clutter of information out there.

Figuring out the healthiest food to eat is harder than learning to use the aptly called smartphone. Supermarkets feature numerous products and it is difficult to navigate through poor health choices to find the foods that are actually *good* for you. More is not better when it comes to the food industry.

Picture this: Standing in the bread aisle, you scratch head, confused. You are trying to be a health-savvy shopper and yet the food industry is not making it easy. Overwhelmed, you allow your child to play the game "eeny meeny miny moe" and *voila*! Little Timmy picks the bread of the week. Without realizing it, you leave the store with the worst kind . . . you know, the "enriched" (more like "depleted") white flour, high fructose corn syrup, fiberless bread that should really be served as your dessert following dinner and not as a sandwich accessory.

Packaged bread is a classic example of a heavily processed food often made with too many unrecognizable and unpronounceable ingredients rather than a basic mixture of real food. This problem is exemplified by the abundance of brands on the market that produce similar poor-quality foods—mimicking more options to the consumer; but in reality, they are all the same, single, unhealthy choice.

Making "choices" like these and not choosing *real* food is one major factor in the rise of obesity in America. It's beyond Houston . . . United States, we have a *big* problem.

A female client, Laura[1], came for an appointment one day with a bag full of empty food packages. An eighty-nine year old woman, Laura was living an organic, real-food way of life for longer than I have been alive. I was helping her gain much-needed weight, despite the painful shadow of irritable bowel syndrome (IBS) lurking in her every bite of food. She was teaching me, too—about *real* food.

One of the plastic food packages she had was for pita, a pocketed flatbread that is a mainstay in my Middle Eastern, Mediterranean culture.

"Beth, I've been buying this bread for weeks and just realized it is not 100 percent whole grain!" Laura exclaimed.

Knowing that she is not one to be taken for a nutritionally uneducated consumer, I examined the package. Unsurprising to me, it was one of the most deceiving food products I have seen. They designed the package to make you think it is the healthiest choice. Here is what was listed on the front of the package:

Organic: Although better for your health in many ways, it does not make a product automatically healthier (see chapter 7).

Wheat Flour: The term makes you think it is whole-wheat flour but it does not say "whole."

100% Natural: The term "natural" is not Food and Drug Administration (FDA) regulated and can mean anything. Petroleum gas is "natural," but would that make us eat it? Also, the 100% at quick glance

---

[1] All names in this book are changed for privacy purposes.

makes you think it was stating "100% whole wheat," a sign I tell my patients to look for on healthier products.

Fat Free, Sugar Free, Fiber Rich: All three are playing on fad diets by highlighting the one nutrient, but is the bread as a whole healthy?

The term *wheat flour* in the ingredients list on the back of the label confirms that this is not, in fact, 100 percent whole wheat. Ultimately, there are better whole-grain choices.

If an educated consumer and nutritionist had to look twice at a brand of Middle Eastern Bakery Pita Bread, what hope is there for those consumers on the run? Most of us go food shopping in a rush, coming from or going to work, with children screaming in the shopping cart. For many of us, food shopping is simply one task on a seemingly endless list of things to do for that specific day. We need food packages to be designed simply, so that if we have only a few seconds to grab bread from the bread aisle, we grab one that will help and not hurt our health.

Wishful thinking? Perhaps. It may be too big of an undertaking to challenge the entire food industry, but *we* can take control over our food choices.

Through this book, I can help make it easier for you to choose foods to eat to create a healthier you. You will receive guidance on how to make your plate, which foods to eat more or less of, how to eat real foods out of your home, and of course, how to shop for real foods. After following the advice in this book, you will notice more energy, a clearer complexion, better digestive health and sleep patterns, and other lifestyle improvements, in addition to the scale sliding downward in the best possible way: continuously, slowly, and steadily.

MY KOSHER SONG

● ● ● ● ● ● ● ● ● ● ● ● ● ● ● ● ● ● ● ●

Along with helping you eat real food for your real life, I will give you a glimpse into my kosher way of life. Food plays an integral role in the

Jewish culture. The importance of family, observance of holidays, and frequent celebrations all share one thing in common: good food.

Born and raised an Orthodox Jew, I am what I call a "mix breed" of both Sephardic (emigrated from Spain to the regions of Aleppo/Damascus Syria and my union with marriage into the Moroccan culture) and Ashkenazi (Russian and Eastern European) ancestry. As a result, my culinary cuisines are eclectic. From savory Middle Eastern and Eastern Mediterranean dishes with spices like cumin and allspice, exotic salads, and kosher Moroccan fish dishes, to classic heart-warming chicken soup, coleslaw and potato salads, I come to you with a tale, and a taste, of two cities.

Traveling back to the days in the old country of my Syrian heritage, the concept of real food was real life. The popular Mediterranean diet was truly a lifestyle. It was frequently quoted for its anti-inflammatory and health-promoting benefits including weight management, improvements in asthma and allergies, decreased risk of Parkinson's disease, rheumatoid arthritis, depression, poor eye health, oral health, and infertility. Families walked to the market bright and early for the best selections, bought their grass-fed meat and fish (delicacies that were typically reserved for Sabbath meals on Friday night and Saturday lunch); purchased local fruits and vegetables and spices just picked from the fields; fermented their own wine, pickles, dairy and cheeses; and cooked their own fresh dishes daily. In fact, Aleppo is frequently referred to as *Haleb*, an Arabic word meaning "He milks." They ate family meals together and took the time to enjoy each other's company and their food.

Most Syrian dishes incorporated vegetables like okra, eggplant, potatoes, mushrooms, and different types of beans, lentils, and peas (see chapter 7). Whole grains, like bulgur, were incorporated into hot and cold dishes (see chapter 6). A variety of salads was also a mainstay in each meal and were heavily seasoned with health-promoting spices (see Recipes). Families fermented and pickled many foods; their own grape leaves, peppers, tomatoes, beets, turnips, cucumbers, and fresh olives soaked in myriad spices. They ate from protein sources that included freshly made cheeses, commonly referred to as Syrian Cheese, and the majority of their dairy intake came from plain cultured yogurt called Laban.

Lastly, the food group with the ominous dark cloud over it today—fats (a true delicacy because it was not readily available and was expensive) was consumed minimally during the Sabbath, but thoroughly enjoyed. Cheryl, the wife of a cancer patient I counseled at the Morris I. Franco Community Cancer Center in Brooklyn, New York, loved her fat. One afternoon, I met with her husband, a seventy-year-old male, Charlie, who had pancreatic cancer. I winced at the diagnosis sprawled in black and white on a form inside his folder. Charlie came to see me after he had completed an intense four-month chemotherapy and radiation cycle that left him both emotionally and physically depleted. He was beginning a seven-week respite and awaiting an update from the doctors on what to do next. It was an opportune time to focus on eating real food.

"Our goal, Charlie," I began to say, "is to build you back up."

He smiled and perked up. Finally, he felt hopeful.

"I know! Look at my legs, I lost all my muscle!" he said with a chuckle. He had a soft-spoken voice and I noticed a foreign twinge to his English.

"What's done is done," I continued to say. "The treatments made you feel the way you do. You can take back control of your life by taking charge of what you eat. Work with what we can control."[2]

I began with my endorsement of proteins and healthy fats. I spoke of how necessary they are to everyone's diet—and how especially critical they were to Charlie's. I could see a sense of understanding come over Cheryl's face as I spoke to her husband. Cheryl was born and raised in Syria on a real-food diet that changed once she moved to America in adulthood.

Cheryl told us about her past diet. She remembered going to the market and paying extra money to buy the fat and bones of the animals. What would now be discarded as scraps were treasures to her family. Her

---

[2] This book is not intended to diagnose, treat, cure, or prevent any disease.

mother cooked the fat and made bone marrow broths. She concluded with what I often hear from immigrants: "And we didn't know about these health problems we hear of today." (Back then they did not suffer many of the health problems of today such as the rapid rise in cancer, allergies and asthma.)

Shocking, right? They were eating what we were told is unhealthy: foods high in fat. Is there something we're missing?

THE MISSING PIECE TO THE HEALTH PUZZLE

There is a piece missing, but it is mostly in *our* puzzle not theirs. It is called real food. To me, *real food* is defined as the closest thing to being fresh and whole, minimally processed, G–d given, and available since biblical times. There are many definitions of "real, whole food" and people regularly debate topics such as "Which foods did the cavemen eat?" and "Is an only plant-based diet the answer?"

Throughout this book, my goal is to fly above the controversies. While I intend to present both sides to every debate, I will explain my takeaway for you to incorporate into your real-food diet with my kosher seal of approval. Here are the foods I fit into the category of "real" for optimal health:

- Grass-fed beef and chicken
- Pastured eggs
- Fermented dairy
- Whole grains
- Plant-based oils

- Nuts
- Seeds
- Fruits
- Vegetables
- Legumes

All preferably organic, all with kosher certification to fit into my real-food kosher diet.

The list encompasses all food groups. Allow me to repeat: *all* food groups. Restriction is never the answer to better health; but the emphasis on *quality* of foods is key. A calorie is no longer thought to be just a calorie. Grass-fed meat ensures the animals are not fed pro-inflammatory soy or corn, makes more vitamin D from the sunlight, and the meat is higher in other fat-soluble vitamins and the anti-inflammatory Omega-3 fatty acids. Quality proteins like pastured eggs can be 20 percent higher in Omega-3 fats. The fermented dairy incorporates enzymes and natural probiotics that feed our gut with disease-fighting bacteria and helps to promote easier digestion and immune health. Aside from reports of better taste, organic produce helps minimize the toxic load on our systems and the environment. Whole grains maintain their nutritional quality of fiber, B vitamins, iron, and minerals like magnesium and selenium—and some even have more protein, too.

A well-balanced diet, with variety, freshness, and satisfying flavor, is not a novel concept, but is one that has gotten lost to controversy. In my path toward better health, I exposed myself to many different nutrition styles. Like a trendy dress, I wore a diet until it was no longer in style and switched to the next one. I fell hard for the different mantras: red meat is evil, all carbohydrates are bad, don't eat all day and eat only at night, then eat all day and not at night. I was left like most of us: confused, exhausted, and gaining weight. I did not feel healthy.

Growing up, I loved all food, especially junk food. As a child, I looked forward to going to dance class after school. My friends and I would arrive at dance class forty-five minutes before it started. The first thing we did was walk five doors down and into a liquor store. Not to drink alcohol, of course, but to buy the snack bags at the register. The eight of us would run a tab and buy one twenty-four ounce bag of chips. I heaved down more than my share, licking each finger as though it would be the last time I would taste that flavor.

In high school, I was introduced to the world of dieting. I witnessed students bringing a salad, a scooped out "bagel," or nothing for lunch, and I heard frequent complaints of being fat. My way of being nutritious was eating pretzels and friends' leftovers for lunch and drinking at least two cans of Dr. Pepper soda during the school day.

I also began to exercise during high school. I tagged along with my father to the gym two nights per week and rewarded myself with a Coca-Cola slurpee afterward. One night as I got my fix and guzzled the slurpee down, I remember my father casually mentioning, "You know, we just put all that hard work into burning calories." The comment set the foundation, in a healthy way.

"Ooohhh," I thought, "it's not only what you push out of your body, but what you put in as well." I was vigorously missing the other half of health—the better half.

It was not until college that I became interested in nutrition as a science. Since I was an English major, I needed special permission from the head of the biology department to take an elective in nutrition. The professor asked quizzically, "Why does an English major want to take a science course?"—a question that followed me throughout my career.

I answered, "Does a scientist not need to know English?" He signed the paper with no further comment. To me, I never saw a conflict.

During that time, I also went on the South Beach Diet and, while I do not support the avoidance of carbohydrates, I learned a lot about the glycemic index and the effects of blood sugar on one's health. The seeds of how food affects the body were now planted in my mind.

Throughout my continuing education for a master's of science degree in nutrition and working in the field as a registered dietitian, I strategically exposed myself to different schools of nutrition thought. From the mainstream to alternative, I worked in a hospital setting, a nursing home, and with children with Attention Deficit Hyperactivity Disorder (ADHD) and autism. I found that each had their own method of treating various diseases from a nutritional perspective. Instead of getting caught up in the controversy, I sought to find the common thread—and I did! I did.

The secret to health—the one nondebatable concept from any medical point-of-view, is a simple message that is subdued by the chaos of what became the world of nutrition:

Eat real food.

What if I were to tell you something brand new hit the market? A miracle drug that can help with weight management, fatigue and trouble sleeping, and managing diseases like diabetes, cancer, IBS, emotional issues of stress and anxiety, in addition to symptoms of autism and ADHD, arthritis, and acne. The cost is low, and it's always available and has no scary side effects. Oh, and it tastes great and comes in different varieties, so if you don't like one, you can try another. Would you be the first person in line to get it?

No need to wait. This miracle is real food!

Throughout the years, we've become a "pill popping" society. And while there is a place for prescriptions when medically necessary, too little emphasis, if any, is placed on the power of food as medicine. One prudent example is in the case of diabetes and the importance of managing blood sugar. Despite medications, blood sugar cannot be adequately controlled without lifestyle improvements in diet and exercise.

CLEANING UP THE DIET: THE FOUNDATION

We can help manage most diseases with the answers to the questions of what, why, when, and how we eat. Our first step is to clean up the diet and replenish your body with nourishing, real foods. The principle is not only what you take out, like the fads of gluten-free, sugar-free, fat-free, or carb-free, but also what foods you add in their places. In short, it is about the diet as a whole—my definition of a whole-foods diet.

Years ago, our ancestors simply ate meat and plants. They physically worked outside all day hunting animals and picking their own grains, fruits, and vegetables.

Hence, problem number one.

Fortunately, the United States provides us with a land of plenty—plenty of opportunities, plenty of comfort, and plenty of ready-made food. The unfortunate part about it is we lost the definition of just that: food. Eating the "whole foods" of biblical days would leave our bodies fully nourished and healthy and our minds clear and focused.

I'm going to take you back to the good old days of eating real food, how G–d meant it to be eaten, and make it fit into your real life. With our small changes, the bigger picture of America will change from one containing an oversized, unhealthy population to one full of fit and fabulous people.

THE KOSHER SEAL: HOW TO READ THIS BOOK

Throughout this book, I will share with you seven steps to living a real life with real food. I will take you inside the different food groups and teach you which ones are better for your health with my "kosher seal" of approval versus foods that are all about the hype or are just plain harmful for your health. I will walk you through the aisles of the supermarket and be your companion when eating outside the home so you can learn to apply the principles of the real-food diet to your real life. Finally, we will end with three weeks of meal plans and some delectable dishes from my own Middle Eastern/Mediterranean–style kitchen to add to your repertoire of simple, healthy, and real-food cuisines.

CHAPTER 2

KOSHER OR NOT KOSHER?

"He humbled you, causing you to hunger and then feeding you with manna, which neither you nor your fathers had known, to teach you that man does not live on bread alone but on every word that comes from the mouth of the lord."

—Deuteronomy 8:3

"And the Lord spoke to Moses and Aaron, saying to them, 'Speak to the people of Israel,' saying, 'These are the living things that you may eat among all the animals that are on the earth. Whatever parts the hoof and is cloven-footed and chews the cud, among the animals, you may eat. Nevertheless, among those that chew the cud or part the hoof, you shall not eat these: The camel, because it chews the cud but does not part the hoof, is unclean to you. And the rock badger, because it chews the cud but does not part the hoof, is unclean to you. . . .'"

—Leviticus 11:1-47

[3]kosher

/'kōSHər/

Adjective

o (of food, or premises in which food is sold, cooked, or eaten) Satisfying the requirements of Jewish law.

o (of a person) Observing Jewish food laws.

Before embarking on your exodus of eating mostly heavily processed foods, it will be helpful to learn about another exodus where more ideal dietary behavior was real life: the days of Moses and the Israelites in the desert.

The foundation of the Israelite, or Jewish, diet is kosher. I used Google.com to find the definition above and was surprised to read the description because it limits the vast scope of the kosher world.

Modern-day vernacular is a more apropos use of the word *kosher*. The meaning extends beyond food and as a reference to anything "pure" or "proper," such as the way to handle a business deal, wear an outfit, or act at work. Aside from kashrut standards (a set of Jewish dietary laws), keeping kosher expands to ways we approach how, when, what, and why we eat, and into how we live a righteous life.

Although kashrut guidelines can be found throughout the days of the forefathers—Abraham, Isaac, and Jacob—they became written law passed from G–d to Moses, the prophet, during the days in the desert. Since then, kosher laws transformed into a huge part of Jewish life and set standards on real food.

THE BIBLE AND REAL FOOD

· ·

We learn many real food, real life lessons from a miracle food in the bible: the manna. After the Israelites were freed as slaves from Egypt under the Pharaoh, G–d provided them with the manna to eat throughout the

---

[3] This book is not meant to be a validated source for kosher laws. Please consult your local rabbinical authority for your individual kosher customs.

forty years traveling through the desert. The manna was described in the Book of Exodus as "a fine, flake-like thing like the frost on the ground and white like the coriander seed in color" (Exodus 16:15). Some commentaries report raw manna tasted like wafers made with oil. Others specify it tasted like honey to children, bread to adults, and oil to the elderly. Israelites also ground manna and pounded it into cakes or baked it, resulting in a flavor of cakes baked in oil.

We can learn from the Israelite's daily routine of collecting the manna quickly from outside their tents before the heat of the sun melted it. They were forbidden to carry the day's portion into the next day. If the manna was left over, it "bred worms and stank."

The exception to the daily collection requirement was in preparation for the Sabbath, day of rest, when they collected double portion to carry over and eat the next day (the introduction of the Sabbath was instituted at that time since you cannot carry anything outside the home on the Sabbath):

> *"This is what the LORD commanded: 'Tomorrow is to be a day of rest, a holy Sabbath to the LORD. So bake what you want to bake and boil what you want to boil. Save whatever is left and keep it until morning." (Exodus 16:23-24)*

If only we can incorporate their dietary habits into ours: eat daily, G–d given, fresh foods gathered from right outside our homes (local farms) for our families to eat.

MANNA AND ME

While I was in elementary school, I remember learning the manna tasted like anything you wanted. I pictured a scene out of the movie *Willie Wonka & the Chocolate Factory* that introduced the "everlasting gobstoppers." If gobstoppers were real, I'd think the manna would have similar qualities. There would be a few interesting limitations: the manna would

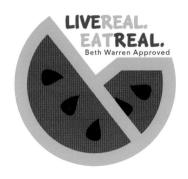

not taste like fish, cucumbers, melons, leeks, onion, or garlic as stated in the book of Bamidbar, 11:5—"We remember the fish, which we were wont to eat in Egypt for nought; the cucumbers, and the melons, and the leeks, and the onions, and the garlic"—because it was thought to be unhealthy for nursing mothers and infants, as Rashi (Rabbi Shlomo Yitzhaki, a medieval French commentator on the Talmud and Tanakh [Hebrew bible]) specified.

The guidelines for living a real kosher life with real food can be traced back to the days in the desert. I stamp my kosher seal on the Israelite way of eating fresh, local foods daily; cooking and preparing what G–d hand-delivered in its natural form. I also approve the potential for food to taste like whatever we can create in our own kitchen. If it is not feasible in your real life to eat this way 100 percent of the time, then aim for 80 percent. It will still have a significant positive impact on your weight and overall health.

How did we lose sight of our G–d intended meal plans?

> **Did you know?**
> The names of both the sugar mannose and its hydrogenated sugar alcohol, mannitol, are derived from manna. By extension, "manna" has been used to refer to any divine or spiritual nourishment.[1]

KASHRUT: THE TECHNICALITITES

Aside from the guidelines of a kosher diet inferring how to eat and how much, it is important to be aware of the stringent technicalities of kashrut.

ANIMAL MEATS

The Bible states that animals are kosher when they both chew their cud and have split hooves (Leviticus 11:3). Kosher animals include cow, ox, lamb, goat, and deer. Having one qualification does not constitute a kosher animal. Specifically, the Bible mentions these unkosher animals: the hare, hyrax, camel, and pig. Unkosher birds are ones that prey, fish-eating water birds, and bats. Kosher fowl are chicken, turkey, duck, goose, pigeon, and pheasant.

In the books of Leviticus and Deuteronomy, we are shown that anything residing in the seas and rivers must have fins and scales to be kosher (Leviticus 11:9). Not kosher fish include catfish, swordfish, skate, sturgeon, monkfish, and mackerel. For the most part, all "flying creeping things," such as shellfish and insects, are not kosher. (There are four exceptions, including locusts.)

The product of any ritually unclean animal is unkosher, such as eggs, jelly, and cheese derived from that source. The same principle applies to kosher animals: their produce such as eggs (without blood present inside), milk, and meat is, for the most part, deemed kosher. There are laws specifically timing when to eat milk versus meat, as well. We also learn not to combine milk with meat from the Bible with this statement in Deuteronomy, 14:21: "You shall not boil a kid in its mother's milk" (see chapter 5).

Cheeses manufactured today must have a *hechsher*, (see Kosher Symbols image) or a kosher certification, since the ingredients call for the enzyme rennet that separates the curds and whey of the dairy to make the cheese. Oftentimes, rennet is derived from the stomach lining of an animal versus microbial and plant sources.

Gelatin, hydrolyzed collagen from the main protein in the connective tissue of animals, is an ingredient with a similar kashrut issue to the rennet in cheese. Since it can be derived from the lining of pigskin, it has to have a kosher certification that shows the gelatin came from a kosher source, i.e. kosher fish skin.

BLOOD

The kashrut laws forbid the consumption of blood because it indicates "the life [being] in the blood." As a result, the meat goes through a process known as *Meliha*. The kosher meat is first soaked in water for a half hour to open its pores. It is heavily salted on both sides and placed on a sloped plank for one hour so that the salt covering draws blood from the meat via osmosis and the blood can drain. Finally, the Shohet (see below) bangs off the salt and rinses the meat three times.

Because there is too much blood in internal organs like livers, lungs, and hearts, these pieces are taken out of the meat before salting for optimal blood removal. However, the hindquarters of nonfowl livestock are strictly

forbidden, unless certain veins and fat deposits are removed. This is a reminder of the time Jacob fought with Esau's guardian angel and was hurt in that area of the body (Genesis 32:33).

Prohibitions against eating pork, shrimp, shellfish, and many types of seafood, most insects, scavenger birds, and various other animals are forbidden in a kosher diet.

RITUAL SLAUGHTER

The process of how to slaughter an animal is paid close attention. The mandatory details were created to ensure the animal dies instantly without unnecessary suffering.

Only a trained professional who is known to be a pious Jew and observes the Sabbath, called a *Shohet*, is allowed to perform the slaughtering process. The large, razor-sharp knife is inspected before each slaughtering to ensure there are no irregularities to circumvent the slaughter. Otherwise, the entire meat will be deemed not kosher.

The Talmud (the body of Jewish civil and ceremonial law and legend comprising the Mishnah [text] and the Gemara [commentary]), later specified laws about the consumption of animals dying from diseases. As a result, the final process after ritual slaughter includes the need for the entire animal meat to be checked to ensure seventy different indicators, such as blemishes or scars, are not present. A blemish may indicate problems with the animal, such as inflammation, which may be passed on to the individual. The final step of checking the meat (especially the lung for any strings attached to it or the slightest hole or scar) is what entitles a cut of meat to be "glatt" kosher, a Yiddish word meaning smooth.

KEEPING KOSHER AND HEALTHY

Being born and bred in the kosher world, I eyewitnessed the evolution of the kosher market. I know that just because a product has a kosher symbol does not mean it is automatically healthier.

Unfortunately, like most aspects of the American diet, the kosher way of life traveled far from its real-food origins of the Israelite days in the desert. Yet, certain kashrut laws place greater emphasis on some foods, like glatt kosher meat, setting them at a higher health caliber than other non-kosher varieties.

Ultimately, the reason why Jewish people keep kosher is simple: because G–d said so. But, the Rambam (Mosheh ben Maimon, called Moses Maimonides, a preeminent medieval Jewish philosopher and one of the most prolific and followed Torah scholars and physicians of the Middle Ages) ventures to share in his book, Guide to the Perplexed (3:48), a surprising theory to explain the rational basis for the Torah's

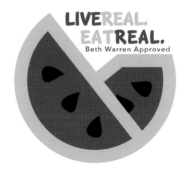

dietary laws: "I maintain that the food which is forbidden by the Law is unwholesome." However, there are modern-day processing methods that have made poor choices out of many inherent kosher, healthier ones.

I stamp my Kosher Seal of Approval on living a kosher life, in general, because it can focus your path toward better health in these ways:

1. **It eliminates about 30 percent of food products from the market and allows you to focus on fewer items to make a more healthful choice.** These days, we are faced with an overwhelming amount of products shadowing healthier choices that only make a smart choice more difficult to make (see chapter 10).

2. Since you are inspecting a food package for kosher ingredients and a *hechsher* (kosher symbol), it encourages you to read food labels.

3. Because of all the laws you read about, keeping kosher also teaches you a sense of discipline when it comes to how to eat and when to eat and acclimates you to saying no to some food choices both inside and outside the home—a practice essential to living a real-food way of real life (see chapter 9).

4. **It is vital to understand that foods with a kosher symbol *do not* make them automatically more healthful.** In the coming chapters, I will show you how to sift through various foods to find the healthy choices amongst kosher real food.

CHAPTER 3

L'CHAIM (TO LIFE)

"G–d, Thou hast appointed me to watch over the life and death of Thy creatures: here am I ready for my vocation."

—*Maimonides, Oath for Physicians*

In the kosher world, it is customary to end a toast with the salute "L'Chaim!" ("To life!") It is common to approach dietary changes with a primary goal of losing weight. During patient assessments, I often find their issues are affecting other areas in addition to their weight. They may not be sleeping well, they may lack energy, feel depressed and anxious, or experience gastrointestinal issues like constipation. You will quickly come to realize through the following chapters that incorporating real foods into your real life surpasses a desire to solely lose weight and allows you to reach the ultimate goal: to have a good and healthy life—a true testament to "L'Chaim." Think: Eat *real* food. Live *real* change.

Heading into any dietary changes with your "I need to be skinny" foot will set you up for long-term failure. Instead, adopt my mantra: "It's not about being skinny or overweight, it's about being healthy." Putting the emphasis on health—a positive message—and *not* the desire to be super skinny lifts an intense pressure that ties too many negative emotions to eating. Any extreme calorie cutting diet would result in weight loss, but does it make you healthier? What you need to make is real-world, lifestyle changes for overall better health, with weight loss as a welcomed corollary.

If you feel overwhelmed as you read on, repeat my mantra. Take comfort in knowing you are not going on another fad diet that is restrictive, temporary, and depressing. Personally, I cringe when I hear patients say the word *diet*. Even though the Greek language interprets diet as simply a way of eating, the word has come to lose its innocence. Nowadays, "dieting" sets off alarm bells in your mind. Your body reacts by going into lockdown mode. I can envision a scene similar to a bank robbery with iron gates crashing down in the vault while overwhelming panic and claustrophobia creeps over you. There is no way the anxious feelings can last for the rest of your life. As a result, whatever restrictive effort you invest is temporary. All the futile hard work leaves you unhappy and unhealthy.

THE REAL-FOOD, REAL-LIFE DIET

I would like to begin by suggesting you obliterate the misconception of the word *diet* from your mind. Instead, we will restore the true terminology as a way of eating by exploring the real foods you should fit into your real life. What that means is that you should aim to eat the way I am going to describe 80 percent of the time. No one is asking for you to be perfect; rather, the goal is to be more mindful of your diet. (Remember, the word *diet* now means "a way of eating"!)

These lifestyle changes pave the way for permanent benefits in not only weight loss, but improvements in energy, mood, sleep, skin, and other areas. Start by taking the pressure off the need to be skinny and instead think about being healthy. You should already feel weight lift off your shoulders.

THE REAL-FOOD DIET FOUNDATION

• • • • • • • • • • • • • • • • • • • •

I will break down my way of eating a real-food diet with these seven simple steps. Think of them as the foundation of the plan—a precursor to more specifics about the actual food choices in the coming chapters. Just as G–d gave Moses the Ten Commandments, I am providing you with my Seven Commandments on how to follow my real-food diet. When in doubt, or in any situation when you are not in control, resort back to these guidelines:

Steps to Living a Real Life with Real Food:

1. Eat real food (minimally processed) about every three hours during the day (no less than two hours after you ate previously, no more than four hours apart).
2. Design your lunch and dinner with the plate model: one-quarter high-quality protein, one-quarter whole grain carbohydrates, and half non-starchy vegetables.
3. For breakfast and snacks, always think protein and fiber.
4. Keep a daily food, hunger, and mood diary.
5. Move it—a minimum of thirty minutes per day!
6. Get six to eight hours of quality sleep per night.
7. Drink up! (Water, that is!)

STEP I: EAT EVERY TWO TO THREE HOURS

Celia, on her first visit, worked with me to map out a meal plan of real food. Her former diet consisted of drinking coffee throughout the day, grabbing a yogurt on occasion, eating dinner, and munching at night. After the meal plan was neatly organized, she looked at it and remarked, "This is a lot of food." Fear set over her and Celia thought she would gain weight as opposed to her goal of losing it.

After beginning to eat the real-food way, Celia realized she was previously falling short of her calorie requirements for the day and overeating at night. Her body was mostly in conservation mode, storing her calories instead of burning them for energy. Celia's metabolism was at a standstill and needed to be revved up by scheduling when to eat.

Despite what you may think about the plan at first, you are not meant to eat more calories than necessary. Rather, you should eat fewer, more nutrient-dense calories in multiple sittings, spread over the course of the day, in a more satisfying and efficient way. You will come to learn the *quality* of food matters in the overall context of *quantity*.

After a few weeks following an eating routine, you will be attuned to, and trusting of, your natural hunger and satiety cues. In fact, the Rambam wrote, "One should eat only when he is hungry and drink only when he's thirsty. . . . One should not eat until his stomach is full but should rather eat around a quarter less than his fill"—an art of eating behavior we will accomplish after beginning an eating schedule.

Imagine this: Your body is like your newborn baby. Here you are, responsible for this precious being, feeling a sense of love and inherent urge to provide for necessities. You would never think of selling it short with foods that are low quality.

Furthermore, a baby thrives on a schedule, just like your body. Your body loves to know when you are going to eat, allowing your metabolism to work at full capacity by trusting that it will get the food it needs on time. Your metabolism is moving, your hormones are balanced—namely insulin (which pulls sugar from the blood and into the cells) and cortisol (the "stress" hormone)—your brain is steadily fueled and you are happy and content, mind and body. If you skip meals, then you fall off schedule, becoming cranky and unhappy like a baby who desperately yearns for consistency, inside and out.

Your goal is to eat about every two to three hours, which helps keep you full and satisfied. Studies show that keeping your insulin hormones in check allows for optimal weight control and health. With breakfast, it is best to start your metabolic clock and eat within one hour of waking. After the natural six- to eight-hour overnight fast while you sleep, your body goes into conservation mode. The opportunity to "clean your internal engine" is welcomed by your body as a break from eating and a time to fulfill other processes including the breaking down of glycogen, the storage form of carbohydrates and, ultimately, fats. As much as we would love to lose fat, remember that fats are also a source of energy in the body (see chapter 4 "Fats: Why We Need Them"). The loss of your body's source for energy, namely glucose, protein, and fats causes the liver to make its own sugar through a process called gluconeogenesis. It is a wonderful survival instinct that ensures your brain is fueled at times of starvation.

Another byproduct of conservation mode is triglycerides, an alternate source of energy when needed. The fat takes advantage of the time without glucose to make as many triglycerides as possible since your body cannot both make triglycerides and take part in the uptake of glucose when you start eating again. The longer you keep your body in starvation mode, the more triglycerides your body creates . . . not a good thing.

Therefore, it is important to stop the starvation process when you wake up on a normal morning so you can begin burning calories, not conserving them. Fueling yourself as fast as possible ignites the fire in your metabolism and provides your muscles with much-needed protein to switch into recovery mode. Otherwise, you will continue breaking down proteins from your muscles so the body can use them. Similar to how a fetus is nourished inside a womb, if you do not supply your body with food, it will get its required nutrients even if it has to pull them from your muscles, bones, vitamin stores, and other places.

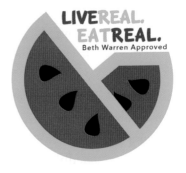

I stamp my Kosher Seal of Approval on starting the real-food diet by eating within one hour of waking up and no more than four hours, no less than two hours, following the previous meal or snack.

REAL-FOOD SNACK ATTACK

Following breakfast, eat a nutritious snack within two to three hours. For example, if you eat breakfast at 8 a.m, then you should eat a snack about 10:30 a.m. A snack is a nutritious power punch that keeps your hormones at bay, your metabolism moving, and palate satisfied. Ideally, it consists of real foods with a protein and fiber combination that fall within the 100–200 calorie range depending on the quality of food and your daily caloric needs (see Snack Ideas). It is not that other snack food options are forbidden, but to encourage your consumption of quality real foods, you are allotted only the one non-real-food snack. For example, if you decide to indulge in a 100-calorie snack pack, then that is all you should consume in that sitting. You shouldn't look for another food to add another 100 calories because those non-real-food calories are metabolized differently than real foods.

The next time to have a snack is between lunch and dinner, along with an optional after-dinner snack if you have a habit of the nighttime munchies. This should always take place within the two- to three- hour window timed from when you ate previously.

Eating at predestined times may feel methodical at the start of living a real life with real food, especially if you are not accustomed to snacking during the day. I have patients that go as far as setting reminders on their smartphones that blink the warning, "Time to eat!" You can also engage a supportive friend to call and verbalize "Eat now." Whatever works for you, staying on top of your eating times is the first step to living a real life with real food. After eating one to two weeks on a schedule, it will begin to feel more habitual and true to your real world, so stick with it!

STEP 2: USE A PLATE MODEL

Being a plate designer is not only for the artsy type. The palette is simple, realistic, and essential to well-balanced, real-food living. The way you fill your plate with food is one method you can control both in and out of your home, so you can always fall back on it (see chapter 9).

How to Make Your Plate

Simply switching from a twelve-inch to a nine-inch plate was shown in a study to reduce your total calorie intake by 20 to 22 percent.[2] Imagine a dotted line dividing the portions on the nine-inch plate: one-quarter lean protein, one-quarter whole grains and starchy vegetables, and half non-starchy vegetables (see My Kosher Plate on the next page). Set the entire plate with each food group and take a minute before eating to soak in the colorful palette, aromatic smells, and anticipation of your meal. This falls in line with a rabbinical mandate to make a blessing to G–d before eating while focusing on the delicious taste, texture, and color of the food. With each bite, chew slowly and put your fork down in between bites. Use the design for both lunch and dinner meals, inside and outside the home. It's that simple. The website www.MYPLATE. gov came up with a similar concept and replaced the more confusing MyPyramid (www.MyPyramid.gov), while the Harvard School of Public Health created one with further specifics on types of food.

The concept of the plate model takes into account multiple nutrition strategies for weight management and better health. Firstly, it balances the food groups, which helps to maintain your blood sugar, factoring in the science of the glycemic index. The array of colorful food groups displayed also ensures you are consuming a variety of nutrients, vitamins, and minerals. Finally, the controlled portions are ensuring you are not overeating since your calories are in check.

I received immediate feedback from patients who were concerned that the size of their regular plates and portions were unquestionably

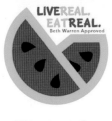

THE KOSHER REAL FOOD PLATE

Use Healthy Oils (like olive oil) for cooking, on salad, and at the table. Limit butter. Avoid Trans Fat.

Drink water, tea or coffee (with little or no sugar). Limit Milk/Dairy (1-2 servings/day) and juice. Avoid sugary drinks.

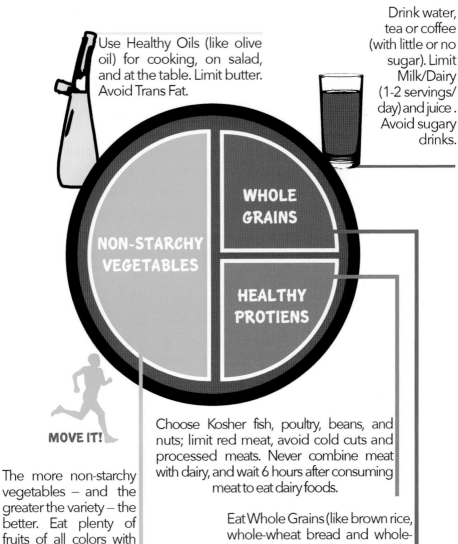

NON-STARCHY VEGETABLES

WHOLE GRAINS

HEALTHY PROTIENS

MOVE IT!

The more non-starchy vegetables – and the greater the variety – the better. Eat plenty of fruits of all colors with snacks.

Choose Kosher fish, poultry, beans, and nuts; limit red meat, avoid cold cuts and processed meats. Never combine meat with dairy, and wait 6 hours after consuming meat to eat dairy foods.

Eat Whole Grains (like brown rice, whole-wheat bread and whole-grain pasta, sprouted when possible). Avoid refined grains (like white rice and white bread).

BASED OFF THE HARVARD SCHOOL OF PUBLIC HEALTH'S "HEALTHY PLATE".

more than this model. They worried about being hungry after eating one plate of food. I advise that if you want to go for a second helping of food, be sure to wait a minimum of twenty minutes. It takes time for your mind to get the hormonal signals from your belly that you are full and satisfied. Cholecystokinin (CCK), for example, increases your sense of fullness during a meal. Leptin is another hormone produced by fat cells that enhances fullness. Leptin is also an adiposity signal that interacts with the brain about the body's needs and satiety, depending on the energy stores. Some research shows leptin amplifies the CCK signals, which amplifies the feeling of fullness. Other studies suggest that leptin also communicates with the neurotransmitter dopamine in the brain to create a feeling of pleasure after eating.

Think about an old-fashioned walky-talky system. You're at one end of the receiver and your friend is running a short distance away, holding the other end of the receiver and waiting for the sound of your voice to come through. It takes time and you need to listen very closely. While waiting after your first plate, sip water, get up from the table, talk to a friend on the phone, enjoy the company of whomever you may be eating with, or keep yourself busy with something else to take your mind off eating. If you are sincerely hungry after the time has elapsed, take more vegetables. Being mindful not to "over-stuff" your stomach at a meal can be traced back to the Talmud, which teaches, "Eat a third, and drink a third, and leave the remaining third of your stomach empty."[3]

There is a way to release the hormone leptin's "stop eating" signals faster from your belly, aside from simply waiting. What I reference is a true miracle worker that actually exists in most real food: fiber. Among a plethora of benefits—including aiding digestion, balancing blood sugar, and helping to lower cholesterol—fiber helps food travel faster to your gut, which triggers the hunger and satiety signals.[4] One of the most studied signals is CCK, which releases a sense of fullness and, there-fore, decreases the size of the meal.[5] The faster those messengers are dispatched, the quicker your brain receives the signal that you are full and satisfied.

Speeding up satiety signals is one reason why I recommend consuming vegetables first, as they are high in fiber. Vegetables also take longer to chew and, therefore, allow more time for your brain to get the satiety message on a second front. Also, vegetables are nutritious and delicious, so you may not want to consume more carbohydrates—the last food group to be eaten off your plate—once your hunger is satisfied. If you consume the food with carbohydrates first, they break down quicker into sugar and do not take as much time to eat, even if you are getting some fiber from your ideal whole-grain options. This helps explain why you may quickly go for a second helping of a refined pasta dish after eating one bowl. Who knew that this order of eating follows a

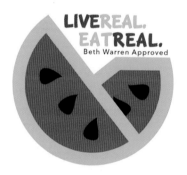

guideline of the Rambam? "One should always begin with the lighter food and finish with the heavier" (Laws of Understanding, 4:2).

I stamp my Kosher Seal of Approval on eating your vegetables first, then protein, and finally starchy foods at each meal on one nine-inch plate.

STEP 3: THE REAL-FOOD COMBINATION

There are fad diets of the past that exploit various food combinations to achieve unfounded claims of weight loss. However, combining foods in line with a concept called the glycemic index (GI) has solid scientific evidence backing its benefits on blood sugar and hormones. The index measures how quickly 100 grams of a food causes a spike and drop in blood sugar. The concept is difficult to implement by its definition alone because there are many factors that affect the GI.

A Real-Food Nosh

A simpler, real-life GI principle you can incorporate into my real-food diet is in the combination of food groups in your meals and snacks. The goal is to balance your blood sugar, hormones, hunger pangs, and weight.

Implementing the plate model in the lunch and dinner design is one way to account for the affect of a food on your blood sugar. Another way to interweave the GI principles into your real-food diet is through your snack design. My ideal snack is a combination of foods with protein and good-quality carbohydrates.

I find many people do not understand what happens when carbohydrates enter the body. Some diets like Atkins and the South Beach Diet, mistakenly declared carbs as evil and advised avoiding them altogether in the short or longterm. Understanding the integral function of carbohydrates inside your body would quickly obliterate these misconceptions.

Foods with carbohydrates start breaking down into sugars, namely glucose, once they enter the mouth; glucose then becomes a supply of your body's primary source of energy. You do not have to consume candy to consume sugars. By eating good-quality carbohydrates, you are giving your body the source of sugar it needs in a healthier way. The word *carbohydrate* is not a stand-alone word to describe a food. It is a chemical property, or nutrient, *in* a food. The accurate way to refer to carbohydrate (commonly called carbs) is through a description of what's in a food. It's more accurate to say that you're eating foods *with* carbohydrates than to say you're eating carbs. Clearing up the definitions of real food in your mind will help pave the way for living *real* change. Carbs are not the weight-loss enemy. On the contrary, foods with carbohydrates are a long-term lifestyle diet savior.

The protein in foods will help your insulin manage the influx of sugar in the blood. Think of the protein as an anchor attached to the sugars in your food, slowing its release. Without the drastic spike and drop in blood sugar after consuming foods, your hormone insulin is able to keep up with the outpouring of sugar and carry it from the blood to your cells to be utilized as energy at a steady, controlled pace. By combining protein with carbohydrates and fiber, your metabolism is running on stress-free cruise control with mini bumps in the road to keep it in check, instead of a hormonal burst slamming on the accelerator, followed by a crash in sheer metabolic exhaustion from the rapid influx of food (see Snack Ideas).

BREAKFAST

The breakfast meal follows the same principles as your snack. The difference is to double your portion of protein. In other words, your snacks are designed as mini meals or half meals.

As mentioned, your body is craving quality protein to replenish its muscle stores when you wake up. Good sources of protein are foods like eggs and legumes (See chapter 7). Foods high in protein also keep you satisfied. As for foods with fiber, they can account for a serving of whole grains or a half a fruit serving: a slice of 100-percent whole-wheat bread or a half-cup of berries are great choices, for example.

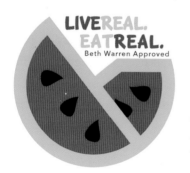

I stamp my Kosher Seal of Approval on choosing high-quality protein and fiber real-food combinations in your snacks and a similar combination, with double the portion of protein, in your breakfast meal.

STEP 4: WRITE IT DOWN!

The clincher at the end of all my consultations is a piece of paper that means more than the words written on it: Food Journal. Typically, the reaction is an involuntary sigh. On top of all the real-food tips you just learned, it may seem difficult to keep a food journal, too. I urge you to write down the answers to these questions about your daily food intake: who, what, when, where, why, and how much?

- Who were you with? Were you eating alone?
- What were you eating?
- Where were you eating? In the car, at home, at your desk, at a restaurant?
- At what time of day was the meal or snack?
- How much of a particular food were you eating at each sitting?
- Why were you eating? Was it because you were hungry or bored?

These questions may seem obvious in a food journal, but I add the columns for mood and hunger scales, as well. Frequently, a passion to lose weight succumbs to pressures and anxieties in your mind. I am commonly presented with patients who want to lose weight and say, "Beth, I know what to do, I just don't do it." Taking into account your mood and hunger during the day can help connect the dots to times you're eating because you're hungry versus when you're eating for other reasons like boredom, stress, or emotional issues.

One way to leap over the barrier of losing weight despite failed attempts in the past or yo-yo dieting is to leap over the hurdles in your mind. By keeping a detailed food and mood journal, we can try to pave a path toward true weight loss and better overall health that goes beyond the food itself.

As much as smartphone applications are helpful, in my practice I find that nothing is better than an old-fashioned pen and paper for your food journaling. It's a great idea to keep notes on your smartphone when you cannot carry your food journal with you, but when you come home in the evening, write it all down and get a true sense of how your day went for both your mind and body. Aside from the mere benefit of painting a clearer picture of your calorie intake and food choices for the day, researchers have proven that people who keep a food journal lose more weight. In a study published in the *American Journal of Preventative Medicine* by Kaiser Permanente Research that studied 1,600 people, researchers found that those who kept a food journal for seven days a

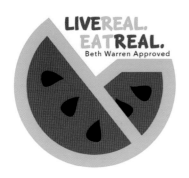

week lost twice as much weight over six months compared to those who were not regular recorders. So get writing!

I stamp my Kosher Seal of Approval on a hand-written food and mood journal or diary, similar to the sample shown on the following page, every day.

STEP 5: MOVE IT!

Picture this: The party night came and you had to do it. You ate that taunting piece of chocolate cake. Now what? Well, the worst thing, despite what you may think, is not that you ate a piece of cake. No one ever became overweight from consuming just a piece of dessert or a teaspoon of sugar. Since we're talking about real life and long term changes, situations like these will happen. Eating the piece of cake becomes a problem when you view the consumption as a "cheat" and a symbolic failure in living a real life with real food. The perception of failure triggers a binge that can take over your real life. The best way to handle these situations is to pick yourself up and move on, knowing with a sense of confidence that you will make a healthier choice next time. Don't think a "cheat" happened, but think "life" happened.

One piece of advice for handling times of indulgences is to move it! Instead of throwing in the towel, take the opportunity to get physically active. Exercise is scientifically proven to boost your mood and benefit your mind, clouding the feelings of guilt you may experience and helping you relax. The Rambam states it point blank, "As long as a person exercises and exerts himself . . . sickness does not befall him and his strength increases . . . . But one who is idle and does not exercise . . . even if he eats healthy foods and maintains healthy habits, all his days will be of ailment and his strength will diminish." Being physically active will give you a fresh start to your day, in addition to the technicality of burning the

DAILY FOOD AND MOOD DIARY

Meal Type	When?	What Food?	How Much?	With Who?	Where?	Hungry Scale 1-10 1-Starving 10-Stuffed	Mood Scale 1-10 1-Sad 10-Happy
Breakfast							
Snack							
Lunch							
Snack							
Dinner							
Snack (optional)							
Fluid Type & Amount							
Move It Minutes: Type & Amount							

*COMPLETE ONE FULL PAGE PER DAY TO REACH YOUR REAL FOOD GOALS.

calories from the one indulgence, and then some. Sustaining muscle not only burns more calories than fat, but also utilizes the hormone insulin and manages glucose more efficiently than fat cells. We build muscles by working out, so get moving!

When I refer to exercise, I may see panic come over a patient's face. Exercise doesn't have to mean an intimidating workout for two hours in a gym setting if that cannot fit into your real life. Think literally: "move it!" Simple ideas such as parking your car farther and walking the rest of the way to work, taking the stairs instead of the elevator, using house cleaning and laundry time as an opportunity to burn some calories, carrying grocery bags to you car, dancing with your children, or carrying a baby around the house when he or she is cranky. All these count toward your "move it" minutes. Seize the opportunities to move any way you can, for as long as you can manage, daily. Set small, attainable goals and when you reach them, push yourself even further. And guess what?

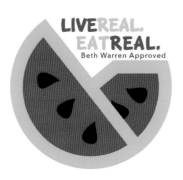

The Rambam similarly defined exercise as "vigorous or gentle movement, or a combination of the two, which increases one's breathing rate," with no mention of gym as a necessity!

I stamp my Kosher Seal of Approval on 30 to 60 minutes of physical activity daily. Two days per week: 30 minutes cardio and 30 minutes resistance training.

STEP 6: SLEEPING BEAUTY

Through studies, inadequate sleep is increasingly shown to affect weight gain. Among other hormones, two specific ones that play a major role in appetite regulation, ghrelin and leptin, are affected by sleep. Ghrelin stimulates appetite and is produced in the gastrointestinal tract, while leptin transmits signals to the brain when you are full. If you do not get an average of six to eight hours of sleep, you alter the balance of these two hormones.

Ghrelin increases and favors obesity and weight gain, increasing your risk of diabetes, high blood pressure, and stroke. A small study had participants sleep eight and a half hours a night for four nights. After one month, participants were asked to sleep four and a half hours per night for four nights, thus resulting in temporary sleep deprivation. They found less insulin sensitivity in those with inadequate sleep, further increasing the risk for diabetes, after just four nights of sleep deprivation![6] You also experience a decrease in leptin the day after a bad night's sleep, so you do not get the signal that you are full and should stop eating. Did you ever feel hungry no matter what you ate the day after sleeping poorly? This explains it!

In a study conducted by the University of Chicago, researchers also found that male participants craved 45 percent more carbohydrates and energy-dense foods when they did not get adequate sleep. A Stanford University study tested one thousand volunteers and found the same hormonal affect in those who slept less than eight hours in addition to a higher percentage of body fat. In the end, all the work you put in trying to live a life with real food can be disrupted if you do not get enough zzz's.

The recommendation of the ideal eight hours of sleep dates back to the Rambam, who also speaks about sleep under the topic of eating right and staying healthy in the Laws of Understanding (4:4): "A day and night together lasts twenty-four hours. It is sufficient that a person sleep one third of that time, which is eight hours. It should be at the end of the night so that there will be from the beginning of his sleep till sunrise eight hours."

STEP 7: DRINK UP!

Hydration plays an important role in weight management. Because the brain's hypothalamus controls the signals for hunger and thirst, sometimes we may eat to placate our thirst, especially since studies suggest that most of our fluid (about 75 percent) comes from our food. One study showed individuals responded "appropriately" by consuming water in response to thirst, in the absence of hunger, only 2 percent of the time. They responded "inappropriately" (i.e., thirsty and hungry but did not drink or eat; not thirsty and not hungry but drank and/or ate; not thirsty but hungry and drank but did not eat; thirsty but not hungry and did not drink but ate) 62 percent of the time.[7]

How Much Fluid?

It is not clear cut how much fluid people need to drink because it depends on each individual's needs (even the Talmud suggests "a flask of water per piece of bread,"[9] to which we are unclear of the measurement today, but clearly indicating a large quantity); for example, how much they sweat, urinate, and consume through foods like fruits and vegetables. Some estimate that women (ages nineteen and older) need 2.7 liters of total fluid per day (more than 11 cups) and men need 3.7 liters (more than 15 cups) per day. Americans drink about two liters of total beverages daily, but less than a quarter of that is water.[10]

We should, therefore, make it a habit to drink fluids, ideally in the form of simple H_2O, to help control dehydration and the risk of trying to appease our thirst with food when we are not hungry. Using data from a national health survey of more than twelve thousand Americans, researchers found that people who drank more plain water tended to eat more fiber, less sugar, and fewer high-calorie foods.[8]

I recommend carrying a water bottle at all times. If it is not constantly with you, you will not drink it. If you are in an office setting, take the opportunity to "move it" by getting up to refill cups of water, killing two "healthy" birds with one stone. Here are some other tips on how to drink more water:

o Add a wedge or slices of fresh fruits or vegetables like lemons, limes, oranges, tangerines, or grapefruit, sliced cucumber, and/or melon.

o Add seasonings like fresh mint leaves, a cinnamon stick, fresh grated ginger root, or fresh grated zest from an organic citrus rind.

o Freeze 100 percent juice and bits of real fruit like berries in ice cube trays to add color and flavor.

OTHER FLUIDS:

Coffee: Sometimes, a patient sneakily covers their cup of coffee as they sit down at my desk and others may guiltily admit they drink it, waiting for my disapproval. Believe it or not, coffee can count toward your fluid requirement. Although many think it acts only as a diuretic, which would dehydrate you, it actually does not cause you to expel more urine than you normally would, though it may have you running to the bathroom a little faster than usual. Also, a cup of coffee is mostly water, so the water consumed in the process of drinking the coffee may offset the diuretic effects. And be sure to remember that any diuretic effect is due to the caffeine in the coffee, so any caffeinated beverage like soda or tea, and even a food like chocolate, will have the same result.

Coffee, about one to three cups per day, can be used on our path toward better health and weight loss. Some of the most interesting studies show that coffee lowers the risk of developing kidney stones, gallstones, and type 2 diabetes and is linked to fewer suicides—most likely due to coffee's ability to act as a mild antidepressant.[11]

Coffee becomes an issue if you have adverse side effects to caffeine (shaking, irritability, and insomnia) or a morning headache if you miss your cup o' joe, so be sure to note any symptoms in your Food and Mood Journal. I also find in my clinical experience that people may use coffee to mask their hunger and sip it constantly throughout the day; which is problematic because it pretty much guarantees you will overeat at your next chow-down time, which is not recommended. Is coffee essential?

No. But if you need a cup or two to get through your day, stop feeling guilty about it!

Tea: Many of the benefits to the caffeine in coffee can be applied to caffeinated teas, as well. More than that, each herbal tea has its own health properties. I strongly urge you to drink teas that aid digestion and may leave you with a flatter tummy like fennel, ginger, mint (or referred to as "Nana" in the Moroccan circles made with real mint leaves), and chamomile, along with green tea. Green tea is unique as it has a marvelous antioxidant called Epigallocatechin gallate (EGCG), which is linked with anti-cancer[12] and anti-inflammatory properties and helps manage weight.[13]

Alcohol: Alcohol in moderation, about one drink per day, seems safe for most people. Dr. Walter Willet explains it may offer protection against heart disease and stroke and may aid in digestion of your meal. I like to promote the drink synonymous with a Mediterranean diet: red wine. The antioxidant resveratrol, found on the skin of red grapes, has demonstrated the ability to protect cells from oxidative damage, promotes vasodilation of blood vessels, inhibits platelet aggregation, and smoothes muscle proliferation. In short, it is anti-inflammatory and decreases the risk of atherosclerosis (hardening of arteries).[14] One caveat though: to go truly Mediterranean, and to follow in accordance with the Rambam's ideas,[15] your red wine should be consumed with a meal. For example, in the Jewish culture, one of the Sabbath blessings before a meal is made over a cup of wine and tasted by each person.

Of course, take caution when consuming any type of alcohol as it disrupts your judgment and sleep and interacts with medications. Avoid when pregnant.

Although each person's fluid needs vary, I stamp my Kosher Seal of Approval on drinking a goal of eight cups of water per day as a general guide to meeting your fluid needs and an overall healthy habit.

THE RESULTS YOU CAN EXPECT

Now that you built the foundation by learning the seven steps to living a real life with real food, here is how you can manage your expectations for change. Basically, the faster you follow consistently, the faster you can revel in the results. The more extreme your diet before, the more results you may see. Healthy weight loss is about one to two pounds per week. Sometimes you may lose three pounds in one week and sometimes your weight may stabilize another week. The important point to remember is that your body is adjusting to the new you. It has to catch up with the changes and rearrange the way it handles what is going on inside, like a tracker that changes course.

Aside from the changes in weight, take note in your food journal about changes in mood, energy, sleep, and stool. The first thing to change by eating a real-food diet is your poop! Also, did your headaches disappear? Are you sleeping better? Do you have more energy? Has your mood improved? Are you less stressed? The answers to all these questions show how eating real food is changing your real life for the better. You will quickly learn that living a real life with real food is not only about the pounds on the scale; it also fulfills a greater goal of feeling and looking healthy.

Another important factor to be on the lookout for is how your clothes are fitting. The scale shows everything: if you ate salty food that day or the day before, if you drank a glass of water, of if you're experiencing hormonal fluctuations. Also, water, which is dense and weighs more than fat, fills into the area of the body where fat is lost. Therefore, you may not notice the numbers on the scale falling drastically, which is a good thing because we are interested in losing fat, not muscle or water. Sometimes a better gauge of results is noticing the loss in inches. Losing visceral fat and improving your waist-to-hip ratio will decrease the risk of developing diseases like diabetes and heart disease. Whatever the beneficial changes you notice, write them down and use them for motivation to continue.

I am excited for you to begin this journey and bask in the glory of living a real life with real food!

Real Life, Real Food, Real Story

Rachel, a patient of mine, needed help. After having three children within six years, Rachel could not get her weight down and shrink what she referred to as her problem area: the hips. Aside from her weight issues, she was experiencing intense migraines, nausea to the point of having dizzy spells, and motion sickness often, along with fatigue. It was difficult for her to keep up with her job and look after her three small children. During the day, she skipped meals, drank coffee, and ate "wacky mac"–type food for dinner for the reasons of convenience, accessibility, and sheer exhaustion. Because of the kosher issues with having to check produce for bugs, she avoided most vegetables. Rachel's diet was severely lacking in protein because she disliked meat and did not know what proteins to substitute.

After adopting the real-food way of life, Rachel incorporated quality proteins from the legume family: beans, lentils, and chickpeas. She also found a way to add more vegetables to her diet, which included a juice made with spinach as a snack. Despite Rachel's hectic life, her chronic migraines disappeared and she met her weight-loss and waist-measurement goals. Rachel's energy improved and she became an overall happier, less-stressed mom and wife. Rachel became such a pro at a real-food life that she started giving *me* tantalizing real-food recipes!

Weight-loss Challenges. I run "Lose Weight, Gain Health, Win Money" challenges. Teaming up with a certified Zumba instructor, Lynda Levy, the goal was to promote lifestyle changes through exercise and a real-food diet. After the Zumba class, once a week for eight weeks, I taught and gave the real-food meal plans and conducted the weigh-ins. The participants developed strategies for eating out and attended supermarket tours on how to shop for real food and recipes. Nutrition education is the key to successful and sustainable weight loss. The winners lost on average 10 pounds and 7.8 inches each. And they kept their real-food principles as a part of their real life: the real gift that keeps on giving.

THE REAL-FOOD DIET

By keeping to my dietary guidelines, you will begin incorporating real-food principles into your real life. They are simple steps on the path to a healthier you at your healthiest weight. Once you master the foundational Seven Commandments, you can progress toward incorporating better-quality food choices. You may refer to the sample meal plans to help wrap your mind around the principles of a real-food diet plan. My goal, however, is to wean you off the meal plans and instill the know-how of making your own quality real-food choices in your real life.

In the coming chapters, I will help guide you toward real-food choices by explaining the importance of quality in each food group. I ardently believe, and bear witness, that through learning about your food, you will make better choices on your own out in the real world. The real-food diet will become a lifestyle and you will be in the driver's seat, always in charge of your food choices without allowing them to be in control of you. Good luck!

YOU ARE WHAT YOU EAT: A DETAILED LOOK INTO REAL FOODS

"For the Lord your G-d is bringing you into a good land
. . . of wheat and barley and grapevines and figs and
pomegranates; a land of olives and honey (from dates)."

—*Deuteronomy 8:7-8*

CHAPTER 4

FAT—THE TRUE DEFINITION

"What is 'the delight of Shabbat'? This refers to the statement of our Sages that a person should prepare especially delicious fatty meat and special wine for Shabbat, according to what he can afford. The more one spends on Shabbat expenses, and the more one prepares tasty foods for this day, the more praiseworthy it is."
—*Rambam, Hilchot Shabbat 30:7*

Walking through the streets, your home, your office, or at an event, you may hear or say, "I feel fat," "That food will make me fat," or "Do these jeans make me look fat?" Like the word *kosher*, the meaning of the word *fat* has come to define different feelings, appearances, and attitudes about ourselves, others, and food. As a result, we have forgotten its real, simple meaning.

I put the search term "Definition of fat," into the Google search engine and a link to Dictionary.com stated:

FAT adjective, fat·ter, fat·test, noun, verb, fat·ted, fat·ting.
adjective

1. having too much flabby tissue; corpulent; obese: a fat person.
2. plump; well-fed: a good, fat chicken.
3. consisting of or containing fat; greasy; oily: fat gravy; fat meat.
4. profitable, as an office: a fat job on the city commission.
5. affording good opportunities, especially for gain: a fat business contract.

Reading through these definitions leaves a bad taste in my mouth. I wouldn't be surprised if you're like the many people who view fat far beyond its molecular definition. But there is a larger problem with using the word *fat* to describe how we feel, see ourselves, see our food, and view others. Simply put, it breeds negative emotions. When we think of fat, we experience fear—a fear of gaining weight, not fitting into a bridesmaid dress for our best friend's wedding, getting picked on by friends or colleagues, and the reason why we cannot find the perfect match and live happily ever after. Ultimately, it makes us afraid of foods with fat in them.

Tying such a strong negative emotion to eating is a big no-no. It places an intense pressure that leads to an unhealthy relationship with food. As a result, you may avoid many foods because you associate them with making you fat, even when there is no fat in the product. (I have been told everything from crackers to cookies with 0 grams of fat are "fattening," to which I counter, "You mean unhealthy? Because there is distinctly 0 grams of fat in this food-like product.")

Perhaps you try so hard to avoid "forbidden fats" that when you eat them, you binge. Either route you take does not make a healthier, skinnier you. By grouping all fats together, it is easier to write them off as evil and then use them as an excuse for your unhealthy ways and unhappiness with your physical appearance.

Avoiding foods with fat has a poor impact on your health and your goals of weight maintenance. There are different kinds of fats; some have the potential to hurt, but some serve a big function to help. In this chapter, I will guide your view of healthy fats in the diet solely as an essential food group that is critical to your body's health and weight-loss success. Oh yeah, and a deliciously satisfying gift from G–d, too!

F-A-T: THE DEFINITION

● ●

Allow me to narrow down the definition of fats in your mind to this: *fat is a nutrient.* Plain and simple. It is not an imagined threat, like a scary monster hiding in your closet, nor should it be an adjective, adverb, or used as any other way of describing anything other than the nutritional content of a food—separate food from your emotion!

Eggs, nuts, seeds, healthy oils like avocado, olive, walnut and flax are all tied to great health benefits.

Of course, too much of a good thing can easily turn into a negative. The quote at the beginning of this chapter from the Rambam emphasizes the importance of enjoying quality fats of meat as part of the biblical commandment to beautify the Sabbath; but that only promotes fat consumption at *one* dinner and *one* lunch meal per week. In the Hebrew language, the word for someone who is overweight (shaman) and oil (shemen) are spelled with the same three letters: shin, mem, and nun. The implication is: if you eat too much oil, you will get fat. A tablespoon of oil will cost you 119 calories from your daily caloric requirements. If you choose quality oil, however, those calories will be well spent.

It is not uncommon for a patient to be living off 100-calorie snack packs prior to seeing me. From Stella D'oro® and Chips Ahoy!® to Entenmenn's® brands, food manufacturers have grabbed the opportunity to package their processed foods in tiny, cute bags and make them appear to be a healthier choice for consumers. How convenient for both them and the buyer: the buyer is happy to have the portion-controlled package to eat on the go, guilt-free, and the manufacturer has sidestepped the opportunity to actually make the food itself healthier and instead simply reduced the size.

As important as portion control is to a healthy diet, the *quality* of food choices is right up there on my hierarchy of health priorities. High-quality foods, like nuts, may have more calories per serving than a 100-calorie snack pack, for example, but the satiating quality of nuts is correlated with making you eat fewer calories in your day, overall, so the calories consumed will be compensated.[16] Some components of nuts are also not completely absorbed by your body, which means some of the calories you consume come out in your poop.

Also, these quality calories, like those in nuts, are filled with nutrients your body needs, typically in its natural form—unlike processed foods, such as Nabisco®'s Oreo® 100-calorie pack, which lists its main ingredients as: dextrose, cornstarch, leavening (baking soda and/or calcium phosphate), color added, salt, vanillin—an artificial flavor. If you're asking yourself "What am I eating? Is this even food?" know that this is the question your body has been asking for as long as you have been eating mostly heavily processed foods. You may finish eating within a few seconds and move on to your next activity, but once you've consumed that food, your body is only beginning the processes of digestion and absorption, setting off a systematic process inside your body. The body has to undergo a different process to break down the chemicals and sift through the nutrients it can use, which slows down your metabolism.

Nuts, seeds, avocados, and other quality calories are filled with nutrients your body loves. Like the diesel of gasoline, these foods are prime and granted VIP access straight through the body, speeding up your resting metabolism. The process of digesting quality calories increases your resting metabolic rate[17] by 11 percent. Your metabolic rate is the burning of calories inside your body as it undergoes its normal processes while you just sit there. (The other two ways to burn calories are through exercise and the thermic effect of food—calories burned while processing and storing foods.)

Another crucial factor is that processed food products are designed to make you eat more. The concept is not a conspiracy theory—it is real! The large amount of salt, sugar, and fat in these products changes brain chemistry the same way an addiction to drugs or gambling can. You become addicted to the food and cannot stop eating, which causes "conditioned hypereating," meaning everytime you even think about a food with fat, sugar,[18] and salt,[19] you cannot help but crave it.[20]

FATS: A HISTORY

● ● ● ● ● ● ● ● ● ● ● ● ● ● ● ● ● ● ● ●

Your feelings of disgust about fat are not your fault. In the early 1990s, we were told all fats are bad. The food industry caught onto the marketing niche and created products to suit the fad of the century. Quickly, we went on a shopping binge for all products that were deemed "fat free." As a child, I remember my pantry filled with fat-free cookies, brownies, and potato chips. I used to stop at the local 7-Eleven to purchase the original "dietetic" tastee-d-lite. *Voila*—eating these foods was supposed to make us magically healthier.

Nothing could have been further from reality. As a result of the low-fat craze, food lost nutritional quality. From ice cream—with the standard ingredients of cream, sugar, and milk—came a chemically designed food-like product with a long list of ingredients you cannot pronounce just to deem it "fat free." Not to mention, fat-free foods taste unappealing and lack satiety and satisfaction factors—the very opposite of what the foods *with* fat are proven to provide.

Take a look at the ingredients for Breyers® Fat Free Creamy Vanilla ice cream: skim milk, sugar, corn syrup, polydextrose, maltodextrin, propylene glycol monoesters, mono and diglycerides, cellulose gum, cream (adds a dietarily insignificant amount of fat), carob bean gum, guar gum, natural flavor, carrageenan, ice structuring protein, vitamin a palmitate, annatto (for color). Sounds appetizing, right?

Products such as Twizzlers® depict my favorite exploitation of the paradoxical fat-free fad: a proud stamp of its idea of health approval—"A Low Fat Food."

I discovered another one of my personal favorite exploitations while out with my children at Luna Park in Coney Island. This shocking "fat-free" ingredient list stated:

Sugar and Artificial Flavors. It contains:

A) Blue #1 – Boo Blue
B) Red #40 – Silly Nilly
C) Red #2 – Jolly Berry, Cherry Berry
D) Red #40 & Yellow #6 – O-Jay
E) Blue #1 & Red #3 – Spookie Frutti
F) Blue #1, Red #3 & Yellow #6 – Bubble Gum
G) Blue #1, Yellow #6 & Green #3 – Leapin' Lime
H) Yellow #5 – Pina Colada, Banana Bonanza
I) Yellow #5 & Blue #1 – Sassy Apple

Did you guess these were the ingredients in cotton candy? I'd like to think that if I hadn't already known what it was, I definitely wouldn't have guessed it based on this list—especially since whatever was written on the package was not edible. (But it was fat free!)

Are you surprised by the fact that the era of a fat-free diet coincided with the rise in obesity? One study, which termed the trend The American Paradox, showed that the prevalence of overweight female and male adults in the United States increased from 25.4 percent between 1976 and 1980 to 33.3 percent between 1988 and 1991—a 31 percent increase. During the same period, average fat intake, adjusted for total calories, dropped from 41 percent to 36.6 percent, an 11 percent decrease. Concurrently, there was a dramatic rise in the percentage of the US population consuming low-calorie products, from 19 percent of the population in 1978 to 76 percent in 1991.

What happened? Did the researchers miss the boat and make the problem worse? It seems that the era picked up on only one piece of the puzzle. While happy to exploit the findings on the dangers of fat to your health, the world did not ask the fundamental questions: Are all fats truly bad? Does taking fat out of a product make us any healthier?

The answer is an emphatic *no*!

I am strategically discussing fats in the first step to living a real life with real food because, in my clinical experience, it is the most difficult factor to reverse in your mind. Although the United States went through many food revolutions, from carb-free to sugar-free, to many other diet headlines, the fat-free frenzy may be lurking in the shadows of your mind. Some patients seemingly listen to me talk about healthy fat options to include in their diets; but instead are distracted with calculating the fat grams of each food I mention. Before you can begin to incorporate other real foods into your real life, you need to accept healthy fats as part of your diet. As you read on, be open-minded to the possibility that consuming more of the *right* fat or "fattening" products, as you may refer to them, will actually aid in your weight-loss and better-health goals!

FATS: WHY DO WE NEED THEM?

1. Fat provides needed energy—9 calories per gram, which is 5 more calories per gram than protein and carbohydrates.
2. Fat helps to extend the duration of exercise. Calories from carbohydrates are used within the first twenty minutes of exercise. After that, fat is broken down for energy.[21]
3. Fats contain essential fatty acids, which are necessary for proper brain function[22] and help in physical performance.[23]
4. Fat is needed so your body can absorb the fat-soluble vitamins A, D, E, and K and thwart these vitamin deficiencies.[24]
5. Fat enhances flavor and texture in foods and prevents them from being dry and bland.[25,26]

6. Fat allows for more satisfaction from foods and prevents hunger soon after meals.[27,28]

7. Fat may help produce endorphins (pleasurable feelings made from these natural substances in your brain).[29]

8. Fats help control cravings since diets too low in fat (less than 20 to 25 percent of total calories) may trigger cravings.[30]

9. Fat makes up hormones, which help to regulate the female menstrual cycle.

10. Fat acts as insulation by filling fat cells (adipose tissue) and protecting you in cold weather (*brrr!*).[31]

11. Fat makes us happier by elevating our mood, resulting in less depression.[32,33]

12. Fat has been shown to:

    o improve cognitive function in the elderly,[34]
    o improve learning and attention span in school children,[35]
    o improve vision, especially night vision,[36]
    o lower the risk of cardiovascular disease,
    o lower the risk of breast and colon cancer,
    o and promote healthy skin and hair.

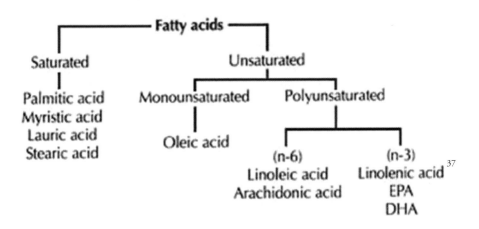

FATS: THE GOOD, THE BAD, AND THE IN-BETWEEN

● ●

Now that we know the real definition of fats and have an idea of their overall function inside our bodies, let us learn about the different kinds and where they can fit into our real life with real food.

MONOUNSATURATED FATS

Monounsaturated fats are classified by the sole double bond on their fatty acid chain. They are liquid at room temperature and transform into semi-solid or solid when refrigerated. Monounsaturated fats may reduce LDL cholesterol ("bad") and lower your risk of stroke and cardiovascular disease.[38] Sources of monounsaturated fats are usually high in vitamin E, which acts as an antioxidant in our bodies and is often low amongst Americans.

The current recommendation is to consume 10 to 15 percent of fats as monounsaturated. Be sure to refrigerate your unsaturated fat sources since they are more vulnerable to rancidity in heat.

Sources of Monounsaturated Fats

Monounsaturated fats are found in natural foods such as high-fat fruits, including green and black olives and avocados.

- o Olive oil is about 75 percent monounsaturated fat.
- o The high-oleic variety sunflower oil contains as much as 85 percent monounsaturated fat.
- o Canola oil and cashews are both about 58 percent monounsaturated fat.

Other sources high in monounsaturated fat include pistachios, peanuts, almonds, hazelnuts, macadamia, pecans, and Brazil nuts along with the aforementioned high-fat fruits.

TRANS FATS

The processed form of trans fat is a major culprit in blocking—literally—our paths toward better health. Hydrogenation, the process of changing liquid oils into semi-solid and solid fats, causes the creation of trans fat. The difference between the processed trans fats and those that are naturally occurring is a simple switch in chemistry that actually causes a big change in function once inside the body:

Because the structure is not crowded, like the "cis" fatty acid that is naturally occurring (second image), it does not bend and, therefore, enzymes and other molecules cannot bind to it. Like trying to use a key in the wrong lock, not only will it not open for you to pass through, but it may also get stuck and cause a bigger problem. As a result, trans fats increase the risk of heart disease and atherosclerosis by dangerously

"Trans" fatty acid

Source: biology.clc.uc.edu.

increasing LDL cholesterol (the lipoprotein that brings cholesterol to your heart) and lowering HDL (the good lipoprotein that takes cholesterol away from the heart and other tissues and back to the liver, where it can be disposed of via the gall bladder).

In fact, the straight design of trans fat enables crystal formation and allows it to be solid at room temperature. Think of the original Crisco® product. It would remain solid even if you tried throwing it across the room at a wall. Now, picture the solid form maintaining its consistency inside your body—inside your arteries.

The warnings of the dangers of trans fats began as early as 1958.[39] But the connection was skewed by the food industry, which applied trans fat dangers to all animal fats. During the 1990s, the Harvard School of Public Health also published warnings on the dangerous connections between ischemic heart disease, high cholesterol, and stroke and trans fat products such as margarines, snack foods, and other hydrogenated oils.[40, 41, 42]

What Does Trans Fat Look Like in Your Diet?

When I ask patients about trans fat, almost all are aware of its health dangers. However, many are consuming products that contain trans fats without even knowing it! A ruling by the Federal Drug Administration (FDA) in 2003 required foods to list trans fat on the Nutrition Facts panel, but did you know that for a product to list no trans fat or "trans fat free" on the label, it can still have up to 0.5 grams of trans fat *per serving* of the product?

The flexibility of what is dictated on the food label and product health claims is one reason why becoming an educated consumer is so important (see chapter 10). Whenever it lists the term *partially hydrogenated* amongst the ingredients, it means there are trans fats in the product, despite the "0 grams" that may be highlighted on the label. Go through your pantry and I bet you find at least one product you once thought was a healthy choice. Now that you're wiser, the words *partially hydrogenated* glare back at you from the ingredient list.

Trans Fat and the Kosher World

The kosher world has a bigger challenge excluding trans fats in products since the main alternative ingredient (butter) is dairy. According to the kashrut laws, you are forbidden to mix meat with milk in one meal. Furthermore, you are required to wait six hours after eating meat to consume dairy. To deem the product "pareve" (not containing dairy or meat ingredients), the kosher food industry features ample recipes that require margarine as a trans fat. We're probably the margarine industry's best customers!

There are other ways to incorporate healthy fats into cooking and baking. First, I find that in most recipes requiring margarine, the margarine can be substituted with heart-healthy oils like olive and canola oil. Also, you can try your hand at coconut oil, which is a solid fat that retains its composition in high heat 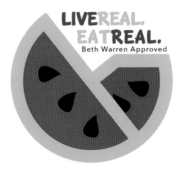 and has more natural properties and health benefits than margarine (see Coconut Oil). The same goes for the use of coconut milk instead of a chemically composed heavy cream in making puddings and other gel-like consistencies.

Tips for Lowering Your Trans Fat Intake

1. Choose liquid vegetable oils or coconut oil instead of margarine and other trans fats or highly processed products.

2. Avoid eating commercially prepared baked goods such as cookies, pies, and donuts, in addition to snack foods, fast foods, and processed foods as much as possible. To be safe, assume that all such products contain trans fats unless "partially hydrogenated" is not listed in the ingredient list *and* the product has 0 grams of trans fat. Fresh food is always best when you have the time to prepare!

3. When foods with partially hydrogenated oils cannot be avoided, choose products that list them near the end of the food label, because it is required for manufacturers to

write the ingredients from the most to the least used in the product. But only use this tip when trapped on an isolated road with a random convenient store as your sole source of food! In other words, always plan ahead with your healthy food choices so this does not happen, but rely on this tip when real life gets the best of you!

CONJUGATED LINOLEIC ACID (CLA)

Conjugated Linoleic Acid (CLA) is a naturally occurring fat that appears in some foods that our bodies do not make. Meat and dairy have the highest forms of CLA, which has been tied to numerous health benefits including:

1. Decreased Cancer Risk

In recent studies, CLA showed promise in fighting breast, lung, and prostate cancers by blocking the three stages of development of cancer cells (initiation, promotion, and progression). Researchers have found non-human subjects who consumed 0.5 percent to 1.5 percent of CLA had experienced 32 percent to 56 percent reduction in benign and malignant tumors.[43]

2. Improved Immune Function

CLA improves immune system function by reducing leukotrienes and prostaglandins, which are responsible for immune system suppression. They may improve allergies by triggering a protective immune system mechanism that blocks the release of IgE antibodies, which is a type of immunoglobulin associated with allergies.[44]

3. Body Fat Management

A study published in the *American Journal of Clinical Nutrition* shows CLA increases lean body mass while reducing overall body fat mass, perhaps as a result of improved insulin sensitivity.[45]

4. Diabetes Prevention and Management

Because of its role in improving insulin sensitivity, CLA can help those with diabetes by improving the movement of glucose into cells, which more efficiently utilizes insulin.[46]

5. Aids in Rheumatoid Arthritis

Because CLA has anti-inflammatory properties, it blocks excess production of pro-inflammatory compounds, such as prostaglandin (PGE2) and cytokines, resulting in less joint damage and inflammation.[47]

6. Heart Disease Prevention

CLA prevents heart disease by lowering bad cholesterol, LDL, and preventing atherosclerosis. The LDL deposits itself in the arteries if there is not enough "good" (HDL) cholesterol to metabolize and take away the LDL cholesterol. When the excess cholesterol and fatty deposits build up, they form plaque in the arteries, which can eventually harden and cause atherosclerosis. Atherosclerosis can lead to serious medical conditions such as a heart attack, embolism, and stroke.[48]

7. Cancer

Animal studies show that as little as 0.5 percent of CLA in your diet could reduce tumors by more than 50 percent, including the following types of cancer: breast, colorectal, lung, skin, and stomach.[49]

Body Composition:

CLA has been beneficial in lowering body fat, with even greater improvement in those who combine exercise with dietary intake of CLA. Animal research has been even more promising, with significant improvements seen in both reducing body fat and in increasing lean body mass.

Previous studies have shown that CLA reduces body fat while preserving muscle tissue. It may also increase your metabolic rate. A study published in the *American Journal of Clinical Nutrition* found that people who took 3.2 grams of CLA a day had a drop in fat mass of about 0.2 pounds a week (that's about one pound a month) compared to those given a placebo.[50]

Food Sources with CLA include:

- High-fat dairy
- Butter
- Egg yolks
- Beef
- Lamb
- Turkey
- Goat
- Linseed oil
- Sunflower oil
- Mushrooms

SATURATED FATS

Saturated fats do not contain any carbon-to-carbon double bonds. Most oils that are solid at room temperature have higher saturated fat content versus liquid oils—notably butter, lard, coconut oil, and cocoa butter. Standard recommendation is that all saturated fats should be limited to 10 percent of the diet of an otherwise healthy individual. Certain kinds and excessive intake of saturated fat may raise LDL and HDL cholesterol levels. (This differs from trans fat, which also lowers HDL and raises LDL even higher.)

SATURATED FATS AND OUR BODY

We do need saturated fats in our bodies. They have important functions such as aiding in the absorption of fat-soluble vitamins and some phytonutrients, building our cell membranes, and being a source of energy. Saturated fats are also important for signaling and stabilization processes in the body.

DIFFERENT FORMS OF SATURATED FATS

Despite what many people believe, there are studies that support the idea that saturated fats can benefit our health. Research conducted in 2013 that reviewed multiple studies showed that dietary saturated fatty acids (SFAs) are not associated with coronary artery disease and other adverse health effects, or worse, are weakly associated in some analyses when other contributing factors, like pro-inflammatory Omega-6 fats (see PUFA), may have had more of an effect.[51] Saturated fats are often grouped under one unhealthy umbrella, so it may come as a surprise that there are different forms with different functions including myristic acid, butyric acid, lauric acid, stearic acid, and palmitic acids.

Myristic Acid

One function of myristic acid is that it stabilizes many different proteins, including those in the immune system that fight tumors. While analyzing phospholipids of a form of white blood cells known as *T-cells* (our bodies' first line of natural defense) from old and young donors, scientists discovered a loss in saturated fats causing age-related declines in white blood cell function. These dysfunctions were corrected when they added myristic and palmitic saturated fatty acids. Myristic acid also plays an important role in cancer prevention and a healthy immune system.[52]

Coconut Oil

One food swept up in controversy is coconut. Typically, the warnings to steer clear of all saturated fats bundle unrefined coconut oil and coconut milk under that umbrella. It is true that they are high in saturated fat, but it is in a different form (medium-chain) than animal fat (long-chain) and other sources. Research has shown that people who eat a lot of coconut in their diets did not have higher blood serum cholesterol or an increased rate of coronary artery disease.[53] Coconuts enhance your body's ability to burn fat and produce ketones, a fuel your brain can use aside from glucose.

Lauric Acid

Lauric acid is also found in coconut and has several functions in the body. For one, it acts as an antimicrobial fatty acid. Its composition is a monoglyceride, which means it is absorbed differently than long-chain fatty acids and, therefore, has fewer heart health risks. Like myristic and palmitic acids, it also helps stabilization when it is attached to certain proteins.[54]

Real Life, Real Food, Real Story

A patient of mine, Laurie, came to see me one summer. She was a cancer survivor who had been cancer-free for five years. Unfortunately, she suffered from post-traumatic stress disorder from her tumultuous ordeal. In an effort to change her unbearable situation, Laurie tried her hand at what she could control—her diet. Based on research done through her own Internet searches, Laurie decided to supplement five tablespoons of coconut oil per day. She would simply dig her tablespoon into the jar and spoon the oil straight into her mouth.

I asked Laurie to bring a copy of her most recent labwork results to our appointment. I took one glance at her report and shockingly remarked, "Laurie, you have the highest HDL cholesterol I've ever seen!" It was then that she informed me of her supplementation habit and how she cut down to three tablespoons after the bloodtest because her total cholesterol was too high as a result.

I was amazed. There are not many ways to increase HDL (exercise is one), and she wasn't doing anything aside from consuming the coconut oil to explain such a high number! (Keep in mind that this is an extreme case of excessive consumption that made her levels out of whack overall, which is not healthy.)

OTHER SATURATED FATS

Stearic acid, found mainly in animal tallows (20–25 percent), is an 18-carbon saturated fatty acid. It is also found in chocolate (about 35 percent). In other foods, it occurs in minor traces of 1 to 2 percent.

The recommendation to consume 10 percent of your fat intake from saturated fat, the mainstream consensus, is disputed within the alternative circles of fat-promoting dieters who argue for as much as 25 percent of fat from saturated sources! According to westonaprice.org, in the 1970s, researchers from Canada tested food fats and found the one with the best proportion of saturated fat was lard, the fat we are told to avoid for fear of grave health consequences!

Regardless of which side you support, fat or less fat for better health, my point is that you should focus on the *quality* of fat. Perhaps this was Cheryl's secret behind the fat consumption of my ancestors (see chapter 1)? I recall memories of my grandmother, who lived until age ninety-one and enjoyed eating real animal fat she pan-fried. Earlier writings

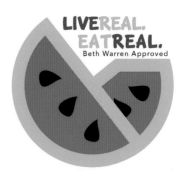

of the Talmud state that fatty meats are good for the whole body.[55] Eating *real* fat amongst the diet of other *real* foods was part of the *real* lives of my past.

Although I am not endorsing saturated fat consumption past 25 percent of your fat intake, I am stressing the importance of quality fat in the diet. Look beyond saturated versus unsaturated and appreciate the functional needs of all kinds of real fat inside our body. Eating fats can be incorporated into Steps Two and Three in my Steps to Living a Real Life with Real Food by adding a teaspoon of foods with healthy fats, like sunflower seeds, to your meal. Another option that falls within the Steps is to add healthy fats that are also high in protein—like nuts, seeds, and avocados—to your meals and snacks, but be sure to keep Step 2 in mind and portion your plate so you do not over-consume calories.

Not all food sources of saturated fat are created equal. For instance, consuming poor-quality foods with saturated fat (like fast-food hamburgers and french fries) encompass more red flags (like excessive calories and trans fats) than benefits. So, stick to real-food choices like the incredible edible egg. (No, not just the whites!) Check out the meal plans at the back of the book for an idea of how to balance fats among other healthful, real-food groups, so you do not over-consume calories.

Real Life, Real Food, Real Story

Aside from the research behind the beneficial effects on healthy fat and our health, I have experienced firsthand the impactful benefits on patients' lives. The most notable account is when I worked with children with autism and attention deficit hyperactivity disorder (ADHD).

Jacob, three years old, was diagnosed with PDD-NOS (Pervasive Developmental Disorder-Not Otherwise Specified) and had difficulty behaving in school, listening to authority, and sitting in one place for more than a few minutes. After lab testing for amino acids, it became clear that Jacob was not metabolizing fats efficiently. He was low in carnitine, which is responsible for shuttling the fats to be used as energy. Instead, it seemed his body was breaking down proteins (specifically branched chain amino acids, leucine, isoleucine, and valine, which were low in the report) from muscle for energy. As a result, he had low muscle tone and was also underweight; his cholesterol, fat-soluble vitamins (notably A and D), along with polyunsaturated acids (see Omega-3 below) were also low.

Aside from other behavioral and medical interventions, Jacob's parents were asked to include more fat in his diet (which at the time consisted of all carbohydrates: pasta, bread, and rice), such as avocados, nuts, seeds, olive and flax oils, coconut oil and meat, along with a supplementation of cod liver oil (with vitamins A and D), Omega-3 fatty acids, and other supplements. Jacob's behavior, muscle tone, and other symptoms improved! Studies are promising in the supplementation of fatty acids, notably Omega-3s, and positive effects on symptoms of ADHD.[56, 57]

For children younger than two years old, the American Academy of Pediatrics (AAP) does not recommend a fat-restricted diet because cholesterol and fat are thought to be important nutrients for brain development. Some who agree with the rationale of the AAP may not agree with the two-year-old age limit. A diet with the right kinds of fat is necessary for continued brain development and essential in children with other medical and developmental issues such as seizures, autism, and ADHD.

POLYUNSATURATED FATS: OMEGA-3 VS OMEGA-6

Two essential fatty acids (EFA), or fats that must be obtained through diet since our bodies do not make them, are the Omega-3 and Omega-6 fatty acids. Both are under the umbrella of polyunsaturated fats and are beneficial in our diets. It is critical that they exist in balance with each other. If you consume too many foods with Omega-6 fats, they make it difficult for Omega-3 absorption because they share the same receptor that allows them to be taken in by our cells.

OMEGA-6

The typical American diet skews the scale heavily on the side of Omega-6 fatty acids fourteen to twenty times![58] The Omega-6 fat, or linoleic acid, is increasingly in the spotlight. One study showed that consumption of dietary linoleic acid in place of saturated fats increased the rates of death from all causes, including coronary heart disease and cardiovascular disease.[59]

Although important to include moderately from real-food sources (see Sources of Omega-6 Fats), excessive consumption of processed foods with Omega-6 fats promotes inflammation inside the body. Chronic inflammation is associated with many disease conditions, including:

- Diabetes
- Heart Disease
- Cancer
- Autism
- ADHD
- Anxiety
- Depression
- Lupus

- Eczema
- Crohn's Disease
- Osteoperosis
- Alzheimers

- Migraines
- Allergies
- Rheumatoid Arthritis
- Obesity

Sources of Omega-6 Fats

- Safflower Oil
- Walnut Oil
- Corn Oil
- Cottonseed Oil
- Soybean Oil

- Sunflower Oil
- Wheat Germ Oil
- Vegetable Oil
- Mayonnaise
- Margarine

OMEGA-3

Your goal with a real-food diet is to skew your scale in favor of Omega-3 fats called linolenic acid. This is also known as an *anti-inflammatory diet*. Aside from the benefits of weight loss and maintenance, it enhances your overall health by lowering your risk of disease conditions. As a result, you feel more energized and less stressed! If there is one trick to reaping the benefits of living a real-food life, consuming anti-inflammatory foods would top the list (see Shopping List, page XX).

Benefits of Omega-3 Fatty Acids[60]

- Stops a buildup of large areas of plaque
- Aids in protection of artery linings by reducing homocysteine and blocking inflammation
- Aids in normal blood pressure maintenance
- Slows formation of blood clots
- Affects response to stress, learning ability, and memory
- Decreases bad cholesterol (LDL) and does not decrease the good (HDL)

- Involved in heartbeat stabilization
- Slows LDL cholesterol from oxidizing

Diets with Omega-3s, specifically DHA, may help form your cell membranes and play a critical role in dictating the functions in your brain cells, since the brain has a high percentage of fat for structural purposes.

Tips For Getting More Omega-3 Fatty Acids into Your Diet

- Use canola oil, flaxseed oil, and other vegetable oils high in Omega-3 fats.
- Remember, the higher the Omega-3 and monounsaturated content of oils, the less they retain their beneficial fatty acids in high heat, such as frying. In fact, they may convert to toxins. Stick to using them in salad dressings, cereals, yogurts, or cooled dishes.
- Choose salmon and other high Omega-3, low-mercury fish and consume at least 7 ounces per week. Prepare fish by grilling, baking, broiling, or poaching. Check out my recipes for more tips.
- Add walnuts or ground flaxseed to cereals, yogurt, and salads. Whole flaxseeds travel through your body undigested.
- Substitute ground flaxseed for fat in baked products. Try using 3 tablespoons of ground flaxseed instead of 1 tablespoon of oil.

FATS AND MY MEDITERRANEAN CULTURE

Consuming foods high in Omega-3 fats, or anti-inflammatory foods, is prominent in my culture. Often referred to as the Mediterranean Diet, this way of eating has consistently been tied to health benefits including weight management, improvements in asthma and allergies, and decreased risk of Parkinson's disease, rheumatoid arthritis, depression, poor eye health, poor oral health, and infertility.

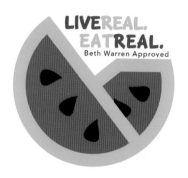

In a fascinating study published in 2013 (the first of its kind), researchers tested 7,400 individuals who were randomly assigned to three different diets. Two were Mediterranean diets enriched with either extra-virgin olive oil or nuts—and other Mediterranean foods—and both included more than seven glasses of wine per week. The control diet was a low-fat diet. Over the course of a few years, many stuck with the guidelines of their diets. Results showed a very significant reduction in death, heart attack, and stroke in the Mediterranean diet groups. The study also proved that one can have seven glasses of red wine or more each week and it might have a favorable effect![61]

We hardly became an obese nation from occasionally eating an egg or having a piece of red meat. The processed, low-quality foods got us here. The overeating and monotonous routine of eating the same poor-quality foods also lead us down this path, not to mention the chronic state of inflammation from the typical American diet (which is heavy in Omega-6 fats) and the obsession of counting calories while being oblivious of what we are really eating. Along the way, we lost what it means to eat real food!

Tips for Choosing the Best Types of Fat

Limit fat in your diet, but don't try to cut it out completely. Focus on reducing foods high in long-chain saturated fat and trans fats and select more foods made with unsaturated fats.

The distinction between the two is simple—and important. The fats you add to your diet should be from natural, fresh, real-food sources. Ingredients like palm oil, coconut oil, butter, and lard may have some beneficial place in our diets if prepared the right way, from the right sources, and in the right proportions.

Consider these tips when making your choices:

o   Sauté with olive oil instead of butter, but only for 1 to 2 minutes, as burning creates carcinogens.

o   Use olive oil in salad dressings and marinades. Use canola oil when baking.

o   Sprinkle slivered nuts or sunflower seeds on salads.

o   Snack on a small handful of nuts rather than potato chips or processed crackers, or try peanut butter or other nut-butter spreads—nonhydrogenated—on celery, bananas, or rice or popcorn cakes.

o   Add slices of avocado, rather than cheese, to your sandwich.

o   Prepare fish, such as salmon, which contains monounsaturated and Omega-3 fats, instead of meat, one or two times a week.

Monounsaturated and polyunsaturated fats have few adverse effects on blood cholesterol levels, but you still need to consume all fats in moderation. Eating large amounts of any fat adds excess calories. Also make sure that fatty foods do not replace more nutritious options, such as fruits, vegetables, legumes, or whole grains.

OH, NUTS! (AND SEEDS!)

Nuts and seeds are written as an option on all my meal plans (unless, of course, you have a nut allergy). In a fourteen-year study of more than 86,000 women participating in the Nurses' Health Study, researchers found that nurses who ate nuts five times a week had fewer instances of heart disease and on average were thinner compared to those who did not eat nuts.[62]

Not only are nuts and seeds great sources of protein, fiber, and anti-oxidant-acting vitamins and minerals like vitamin E and selenium, but they are also proven to aid in weight loss, improve cholesterol levels, and keep you full and satisfied so you eat less throughout your day. The trick is to know how much to eat at one time and how to prepare them. So, put down those caramel-roasted clusters and grab the small, delicious handful of raw almonds while reading these five benefits of incorporating nuts and seeds into your real life with real food:

FIVE BENEFITS OF NUTS AND SEEDS

1. Protein Plant Powerhouse

The American Cancer Association for the prevention of cardiovascular disease and cancer recommends eating a mostly plant-based diet and an ounce of nuts provides about six grams of protein.

2. Source of Healthy Fat

Those great monounsaturated and polyunsaturated fats we discussed as essential to managing inflammation and maintaining the structure of your cells are found in nuts and seeds. People who consumed nuts five times a week had a 35 percent reduction in heart disease risk, according to a *British Medical Journal* study in 1998.

3. Energy-Filled Effects

Because of the high-quality calories, nuts are actually proven to increase your resting metabolism (the kind that is working while you sit and read this book) by 11 percent! They are filled with calories; for example, a single ounce of Brazil nuts contains about 190 calories, so you do need to be mindful of the amount at one time if your goal is weight loss.

Rule of thumb for weight loss: 100–200 calories for snack and about 300–400 calories per meal, depending on your caloric needs. A KIND bar is a great choice for a snack or meal on the run, if needed, because it is portion-controlled and simply incorporates nuts and fruits in one bar, with different variations to consume different benefits.

4. Powerful Minerals

The minerals magnesium, zinc, calcium, and phosphorus, which are needed for bone development, immunity, and energy production, can be found in nuts and seeds. A study of almost four hundred men (ages 45–92) published in the *American Journal of Clinical Nutrition* found a correlation between low blood levels and dietary intake of zinc with osteoporosis at the hip and spine.[63]

5. Natural Vitamins

Nuts and seeds are great sources of vitamins B and E, which help with absorbing protein, maintaining brain health, and boosting our immune system.

Did you know the US Food and Drug Administration has approved a health claim for food labels? It states: "Eating 1.5 ounces per day of most nuts as part of a diet low in saturated fat and cholesterol may reduce the risk of heart disease." These nuts include almonds, hazelnuts, peanuts, pecans, some pine nuts, pistachios, and walnuts—which contain less than 4 grams of saturated fat for a 50-gram (about 1.5 ounces) serving.

Sprouted Nuts

Some people who have nut sensitivities may benefit from sprouting their nuts. Raw, unsprouted nuts have enzyme inhibitors that make them difficult to digest. When the nut sprouts, these inhibitors are deactivated. To begin the sprouting process, all you have to do is soak the nuts overnight in water (about 3–12 hours). Actually, squirrels use the sprouting method by burying their nuts and digging them up when the sensors in their noses identify the nuts have sprouted. High heat from roasting also removes the enzyme inhibitors, but it takes away many of the vitamins and minerals.

SPOTLIGHT ON ALMONDS AND WALNUTS

Almonds:

Who knew? A recent study by the USDA revealed almonds as a rich source of vitamin E that have 20 percent fewer calories than previously thought. In a study published in the April 2002 *Journal of Nutrition*, scientists replaced half of their participants' fat intake with almonds for six weeks. Researchers found that the almond eaters' bad cholesterol went down 6 percent and good cholesterol went up 6 percent. In addition, blood fat dropped 14 percent.

These studies show that a combination of monounsaturated fats and protective plant compounds in nuts known as flavonoids reduces the risk of heart disease.

According to research conducted at the University of Toronto, eating heart-healthy foods, including almonds, can help reduce LDL (bad cholesterol levels) as much as a first-line statin drug.

Research at Tufts University found the flavonoids in almond skins work in synergy with vitamin E to protect artery walls from damage reducing the risk of heart disease.

Walnuts:

Walnuts are unique because they are the only nut that contains a significant amount of alpha-linolenic acid (ALA), the plant-based source of Omega-3 fatty acids. And, according to a 2011 study published in the journal *Food and Function*, the antioxidants in walnuts rank higher in terms of quality and quantity than any other nut.[64]

What is a Serving Size of Nuts?

A serving size of nuts is 30 grams (about 1 ounce). Pistachios have 49 kernels in each serving. Comparatively, almonds have 23; hazelnuts 21; cashews 18; pecans 19; walnuts 14; macadamias 10–12. For the purposes of a real-food snack, you may consume ½ ounce of any form of nut as your protein portion.

SUPERNUTRIENT SEEDS

Thankfully, seeds are growing in popularity. The purchase of hemp seeds, alone, grew 156 percent between 2008 and 2010. Seeds deliver as much protein as nuts (and more, in some cases) and deliver heart-healthy PUFA alpha-linolenic acid (ALA), the plant-based Omega-3 fat also found in walnuts.

There are so many health advantages to seeds that I like to think of them as "vitamins" for their nutritious boost on our paths toward better health. Seeds are rich in fiber, selenium, and vitamin E and are good sources of protein, zinc, and iron. Feel free to sprinkle about a teaspoon on salads and in soups, casseroles, smoothies, muffins, yogurt, granola, cereals, and oatmeal. You can also include more seeds as the protein portion of your snack. Dive into the classic Middle Eastern dip Tehina, which is made from sesame seeds. Be sure to pair it with cucumbers!

HEMP SEEDS

With similar taste and versatility to sunflower seeds, hemp seeds can be eaten raw, toasted, sprinkled on yogurt or salads, or ground into seed butter.

> Hemp Seeds (per tbsp): 4 g protein, 16% daily value for phosphorus, 16% daily value for magnesium, 1 g Omega-3s.

FLAXSEED

Flax is referred to in the biblical text multiple times because it was used most commonly to make linens. But the health benefits of eating flax in all forms are substantial. Flax delivers more ALA than any other plant food. Because your body cannot digest whole flaxseeds, purchase them "milled" or grind seeds in your (clean) coffee grinder or food processor before adding to baked goods or sprinkling over cereal. You can also mix flaxseed oil into salad dressings, breading, or smoothies.

Did you know flaxseeds could help curb hot flashes? The lignins in flax offer a "natural," less potent estrogen effect on hot flashes than the controversial and potentially harmful synthetic hormone therapy.

> Flaxseeds (per tbsp): 2 g protein, 3 g fiber, 13% daily value for manganese, 2 g Omega-3s.

CHIA SEEDS

Chia seeds absorb liquid easily, transforming into a gel-like consistency and making a creamy addition to oats and pancakes while remaining neutral in flavor. The easy absorption allows chia seeds to help sensitive stomachs, whereas flax may be harder to digest because of the lignins. Adding just two tablespoons of chia seeds to your daily diet contributes about 7 grams of fiber, 4 grams of protein, 205 milligrams of calcium, and 5 grams of Omega-3. A mere 3½ tablespoons contains as much Omega-3s as a 32-ounce piece of salmon, but in the plant-based form of ALA (see chapter 8).

The types of fiber in chia are both soluble and insoluble, which explains why the seeds expand in liquids without losing any fiber content.

Aside from helping glycemic control and aiding in diabetes management, chia loading may be even better than carbohydrates or energy drinks to enhance athletic performances for endurance events. Research has also demonstrated that the beneficial effects of Omega-3, as found in chia, has helped those suffering with mood disorders. A meta-analysis of trials involving patients with major depressive disorder and bipolar disorder provided evidence that the Omega-3s in chia reduces symptoms of depression.[65]

> Chia Seeds (per tbsp): 2 g protein, 4 g fiber, 1.75 g Omega-3s

SESAME SEEDS

As the foundation of my favorite dip, Tehina, sesame seeds are a great source of the monounsaturated fatty acid oleic acid, which contains up to 50 percent fatty acids. Sesamol and sesaminol are unique phenolic antioxidants found in sesame seeds. Together, these compounds help combat harmful free radicals from our bodies. They are also a rich source of B-complex vitamins niacin, folic acid, thiamin (vitamin B1), pyridox- ine (vitamin B6), and riboflavin. The minerals calcium, iron, manganese, zinc, magnesium, selenium, and copper are especially concentrated in sesame seeds. Many of these minerals have a vital role in bone mineraliza- tion, red blood cell production, enzyme synthesis, and hormone produc- tion, as well as regulation of cardiac and skeletal muscle activities.

Sesame Seeds (per tbsp): 1.6 g protein, 1.1 g fiber, .05 g Omega-3

SUNFLOWER SEEDS

Often a "munchie" in the Middle Eastern diet, sunflower seeds are a rich source of vitamin B6, which makes antibodies that are needed to fight many diseases, maintain normal nerve function, and make hemoglobin, which carries oxygen in the red blood cells to the tissues. A vitamin B6 deficiency can cause a form of anemia. The more protein you eat, the more vitamin B6 you need to absorb it. We cannot store B6 in our bod- ies, so we have to frequently eat foods with this essential vitamin.

Sunflower Seeds (per tbsp): 1.5 g protein, .9 g fiber, .05 g Omega-3

PUMPKIN SEEDS

A frequent "go-to" after Sabbath meals, pumpkin seeds, referred to as "biz- ard," are often consumed from their shells. They are a rich source of zinc, which supports your immune system and is essential for DNA synthesis and wound healing. Zinc also supports healthy growth and development, especially during pregnancy, in addition to regulating your taste buds—so if things just don't taste right, check your zinc levels!

Pumpkin Seeds (per tbsp): 3.5 g protein, .56 fiber, .05 g Omega-3

Selection and Storage of Seeds

Place seeds in sealed jars, bags, or containers to help ensure freshness. Because seeds are high in fat, they spoil easily. Store them in cool, dark, and dry locations. Seeds can be refrigerated from two months to a year or kept in the freezer for up to two years.

NUTRITION INFORMATION OF SEEDS:

Seed Type (¼ cup)	Calories	Fat (grams)	Fiber (grams)	Protein (grams)
Flaxseed	224	18	12	8
Hemp seeds	162	10	1	11
Pumpkin & Squash seeds in shell, roasted	71	3	4	3
Pumpkin & Squash seeds, roasted	71	3	0	3
Safflower seeds, roasted	130	10	2	4
Sesame seeds in shell, roasted	141	12	3	4
Sesame seeds, roasted	182	15	6	6
Sunflower seeds, roasted	207	19	4	6

Source: Sparkspeople.com

CHAPTER 5

MILK + MEAT: A PREDESTINED MATCH OR AN UNFAITHFUL UNION?

"Then he took curds and milk and the calf that he had prepared,
and set it before them. And he stood by them under the tree
while they ate."

—*Genesis 18:8*

When Abraham was resting after his circumcision, he yearned to host guests. G–d sent him what appeared to be three Ishmaelim men, and Abraham fed them milk and meat.

Commentators clarify that because of the biblical prohibition to consume milk with meat (even though Abraham lived prior to the time G–d gave the Israelites the Torah), the two could not have been served together and, instead, he likely served the dairy first and then the calf meat.

Whenever I think about meat and dairy, my mind wanders to a song by a popular Jewish children's singer, Uncle Moishy. The lyrics are, "And we must never, never, never eat milk and meat together, so join us and sing the kosher song" (sung in the tune of, "John Jacob Jingleheimer Schmidt.") The prohibition against eating milk with meat is one of the sacred laws of kashrut taught from a young age. The source comes from a scripture in the Book of Exodus stating the prohibition of "[b]oiling a (kid) goat in its mother's milk."

From there, the Rambam described that it is forbidden to not only consume milk with meat at the same meal, but one should wait a minimum of six hours after consuming meat to eat dairy because that is how long it takes for the meat to be removed from one's teeth.[66] If one should eat dairy first, he or she must wash out his mouth before consuming meat products.

Because of the stringent laws pertaining to the consumption of the meat and milk food groups, you may think that perhaps they are not meant to be part of a kosher real-food diet. In fact, there are many biblical references supporting both food groups in our diet, but perhaps not in the way you may think.

MEAT AND THE KOSHER DIET:

• •

Aside from the kashrut laws around meat (see chapter 2), eating animals is viewed as a G–d-given right. After the flood during Noah's time, the quality of food—and man's health, for that matter—changed. G–d told Noah, "Every creature that is alive shall be yours to eat. I give them to you as I did the green plants" (Genesis 9:3).

Additionally, meat sacrifices were often required throughout the early days of the Bible. During the first Passover, in the Book of Exodus, the blood of a lamb sacrifice was necessary to save the firstborn sons. If the Israelites did not consume the flesh of the lamb, they would not be protected. During the Sabbath, it is required to consume meat with each meal, both for Friday night dinner and Sabbath lunch.

HERBIVORE VERSUS CARNIVORE

Aside from manna, other biblical references to food groups showed there was more to the Israelite's kosher, real-food diet during the desert travels. At some point, the Israelites complained to Moses for meat. As a result, G–d sent them enough quail to last for months. The delivery resulted in a "quail frenzy": "And the people rose all that day, and all night, and all the following day, and gathered the quail"—some say for thirty-six hours straight (Numbers 11:32)! Many gathered the quail greedily and gluttonously consumed it "[w]hile the meat was still between their teeth, before it was chewed." As a result, G–d was angry: "The anger of the Lord was kindled against the people" (Numbers 11:33). As punishment, those who ate the quail became nauseated and were killed by a plague. This scenario has led to many commentaries on the subject.

G–d provided quail in response to the Israelites' request to eat meat. When the meat was *ravenously consumed*, their bodies became sick and they died. My kosher seal is stamped on consumption of quality red meat *in moderation* and balanced with other food groups.

MEAT AND YOUR HEALTH

Different studies support the overconsumption of red meat and an increased risk of health problems like heart disease and some types of cancers. Conversely, consuming a large proportion of your meals from plant-based sources shows

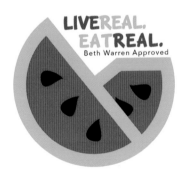

numerous advantages. However, evidence does exist that supports health benefits of meat, when eaten in moderation. The one caveat depends on how the cow was raised.

If a cow is raised in a feedlot, it most likely never sees sunlight and practically lives in manure. The environment breeds bad bacteria, like E. Coli 0157:H7, that can contaminate the cow's meat and have the potential to kill whomever consumes it. Diseases spread like wild fire from cow to cow with conditions such as acidosis, liver abscesses, or feedlot polio, which produces the enzyme thiaminase that destroys vitamin B1, starves the brain of the cow, and creates paralysis.[67] Make no mistake that these cows are sick, really sick. As a result of disease and infection, the cow may receive antibiotics. But that's not all that may be injected; hormones are given to increase its size despite the excessive corn and soy, which already promotes chronic inflammation, fed to the cow for growth. Sounds appetizing, right?

This artificial breeding ground is not the way cows were raised in the olden days. We do not have to go as far back as the biblical days to see this. Instead, we can simply look at the days in Halab, Syria, when my great-grandparents woke up early to buy fresh meat brought to the market from nearby farms, and cooked it for their Sabbath meals. One of my biggest issues with red meat stems from the fact that it comes from cows raised in feedlots and not from the "real cows" meant to graze on green pastures and eat grass. A great documentary that goes into more detail on the farming of cows is *Food, Inc.*

GRASS-FED BEEF

The healthiest and safest way to consume meat is to find the grass-fed variety. Not to be confused with "organic" beef, grass-fed cows literally graze the pastures and eat real grass. Grass, the food cows are meant to eat, also balances the ratio of healthy bacteria in the gut, making the invasion of bad bacteria (like dangerous strains of E. Coli) less likely. As a result of grazing, cows are exposed to sunlight, which allows for the production of more fat-soluble vitamins like A and D along with three to five times more of the essential fatty acid CLA (see chapter 4).[68] In short, their entire genetic makeup is different and you are consuming their meat. It's a cliché, but true: you are what you eat.

THE KOSHER MEAT WORLD

Unfortunately, there are few glatt kosher distributers of grass-fed meat, which makes the price point much higher. Also, some packages list the products as "grain-finished," which means that before slaughter, the farmers feed grass-fed cows grains to increase their size. You cannot be sure what proportion of their feed throughout their lives was really from grass or grain.

Eagerly, I await the shipment of grass-fed meat to my butcher. Since it is not easy to find (sometimes it's in the freezer section), I buy larger amounts and freeze it for my Sabbath meals. Online vendors like Grow and Behold Kosher and KolFoods.com sell grass-fed beef, but be sure to check with your rabbinical authority on finding the right meat sources that fit with your customary kashrut guidelines. Most are not beit yosef, an added stringency necessary for Sephardic customs. The reality is we need more 100 percent grass-fed, glatt kosher, beit yosef farms!

Grass-fed poultry is an easier animal protein to find on the kosher market—and a good thing, too. Chicken is filled with mood-boosting tryptophan and niacin that can decrease your risk of cognitive decline. Tryptophan is also the amino acid that converts into the neurotransmitter melatonin, which helps you sleep better.

I suggest you keep your red meat intake to about two times per week, the equivalent of the Sabbath mealtimes, regardless of farming methods. Remember, each red meat portion should be 3 ounces and only account for one-quarter of your nine-inch plate, but poultry can be 4 ounces (see chapter 3).

Grass-Fed versus Grain-Fed Beef

Research conducted by the USDA and Clemson University in 2009 identified a total of ten areas where grass-fed beef was better than grain-fed beef.[69] They found grass-fed beef was lower in total fat and had higher levels of beta-carotene, vitamin E, the B vitamins thiamin and riboflavin, and the minerals calcium, magnesium, and potassium. The grass-fed meat also had better flavor, color, and texture.

As for quality of fat, grass-fed beef was found to have a better ratio of Omega-6 to Omega-3 fatty acids (1.65 to 4.84) versus 5-to-1 or 13-to-1 in conventional raised cows, along with a higher CLA content, a potential cancer fighter, and vaccenic acid, which can convert into CLA. It is also lower in the saturated fats linked with heart disease. Finally, it my help your weight-loss goals by containing fewer calories. By switching to lean grass-fed beef, the average person in the United States could reduce intake up to an estimated seventeen thousand calories a year, which is equal to losing about five pounds!

DAIRY

*"And when the Lord brings you into the land of the Canaanites,
the Hittites, the Amorites, the Hivites, and the Jebusites, which
he swore to your fathers to give you, a land flowing with milk
and honey, you shall keep this service in this month."*
—*Exodus 13:5*

A primary reference to milk is in the bible when G–d refers to the land of Israel as the "land flowing with milk and honey." At first glance, one would assume "milk" alludes to "cow's milk." However, some commentaries explain the type refers to "goat's milk." Should we take a hint from the text and choose other sources of non-cow's milk?

Dairy is a food group that cannot escape controversy in the modern world. From popular figures in the mainstream nutrition world (such as Dr. Walter Willet, the chair of the department of nutrition in the Harvard School of Public Health and the second-most cited scientist in clinical medicine), to leaders recognizing a link between a dairy intolerance and autism, to those promoting dairy consumption (like the National Dairy Council), the answer about whether we need dairy in our diets comes down to this: it depends who you ask.

Dairy Milk, per cup, skim: 86 calories, 0 g fat, 12 g sugar, 0 g fiber, 8 g protein

The website myplate.gov highlights the benefits of consuming dairy, such as improved bone health (which reduces the risk of osteoporosis), reduced risk of cardiovascular disease, Type 2 diabetes, and high blood pressure, and a good source of nutrients, including calcium (needed for building bones and teeth and maintaining bone mass), potassium (which helps regulate blood pressure), and vitamin D.

One major disputed health claim is dairy's calcium connection with bone health. The bigger question is that even though cow's milk accounts for 75 percent of calcium in the American diet, has it become essential?

Dr. Walter Willet was quoted saying:

"It is not clear how much calcium people need. Worldwide, consumption varies, and countries with average higher calcium intake tend to have higher rates of hip fractures. There is little proof that boosting calcium to currently recommended levels will prevent fractures, the principal complication of osteoporosis, the 'brittle bones' disease, which is found mostly in older women. . . . There is some evidence that high levels of calcium may be associated with prostate and ovarian cancers."[70]

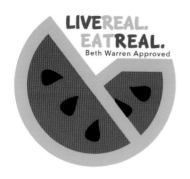

Looking at the research behind both sides of the dairy debate, there may be benefits behind its consumption for those who tolerate cow's milk, but choosing all your protein from dairy and, therefore, consuming too much, is not necessary and may be harmful in different aspects of your health.

A DAIRY INTOLERANCE

Does milk "Do a body good?" as the Dairy Farmers of America's mantra during the 1980s tried to make us believe? In 2007, they reported sales of $11 billion. Whatever the answer, the marketing of the dairy industry obviously worked.

The evidence is mounting, however, on the growing allergy and intolerance to cow's milk. It is reported that about 75 percent of Americans suffer from lactose intolerance. Lactose is the disaccharide in milk made up of galactose and glucose. It requires the secretion from the gut of the enzyme lactase to break down the sugar and digest it. Research shows that after infancy, the amount of the lactase enzyme begins to decrease over time, so the difficulty in digesting dairy increases.

Cow's Milk Allergy versus Intolerance
Keep in mind that a cow's milk allergy is due to a protein allergen, namely the Alpha S1 Casein (it is 80 percent casein and 20 percent whey protein), while lactose intolerance is a consequence of carbohydrate sensitivity.

Aside from a lactase deficiency, there are other reasons behind lactose intolerance. Lactase secretion relies on a healthy gut. If you have gut inflammation, you are not adequately digesting some foods because enzymes are not utilized efficiently to break down a multiple-bond sugar like lactose. Gut inflammation is apparent in cases of Irritable Bowel Syndrome (IBS), in which a dairy intolerance is reported in most cases,[71] along with conditions such as celiac disease and autism spectrum disorders in children.

Because of the intolerance, people with these medical conditions avoid dairy. Most often, they report a cessation of symptoms associated with dairy intolerance including:

o Gastro-intestinal: diarrhea, constipation, IBS, stomach bloating
o Depression and anxiety
o Weight gain or unexplained weight loss
o Respiratory disorders like coughing, asthma, bronchitis, snoring, and sleep apnea
o Sinus pain and headache
o Chronic fatigue or lethargy or lack of motivation
o Skin disorders like eczema, hives, or unexplained rashes
o Stressed immune system: ear infections, colds and flu, bronchitis, yeast infections e.g. thrush

How to Identify an Intolerance

If you want to identify a dairy intolerance, perform an elimination diet under the care of a qualified dietitian and see if symptoms subside. With dairy, you should notice some kind of change within two weeks. To truly answer the question of an intolerance, eliminate soy at first because the soy protein looks similar to dairy and can "trick" the body (see Non-Dairy Sources of Milk).

Real Life, Real Food, Real Story

Jack came to my office complaining of incapacitating abdominal pain that was affecting his daily life. He was severely constipated no matter what he ate. Actually, eating made him feel worse. As a result, he was avoiding all food. Being overweight, he felt content with the fact that he lost twenty pounds in three months since receiving a diagnosis of IBS. Eating nothing, however, still did not help his IBS symptoms.

Through our discussion, Jack agreed that although we both supported him achieving a healthy weight, it was not to be a consequence of not eating real food. Jack left with his "health homework," which was to keep a detailed food diary tracking any symptoms he felt after eating a specific food. Our goal was to decrease Jack's overall gut inflammation by identifying his intolerable foods. We focused on adding anti-inflammatory foods, like healthy fats and nuts, with additional fiber to help his constipation.

Jack came back to see me a quick three weeks later a new man. He walked in confidently and lively. He found that living dairy-free and gluten-free (as we discovered after analyzing his self-made adjustments based on adverse symptoms after eating those foods), significantly eliminated his constipation. As a result, he felt confident incorporating more anti-inflammatory foods into his diet; he was relieved and more social. In those weeks, he lost two "healthy" pounds and is on his way to living a healthier life with real food.

Although there are standard recommendations around IBS, it is difficult to generalize food tolerances. Patients affected may experience yo-yo symptoms such as constipation versus diarrhea in different situations, making it even more critical to keep a food and mood diary (see Food and Mood Diary) to follow your individual reactions to foods.

DAIRY OF MY ANCESTORS

Aside from the evident intolerance many people have to dairy, it is important to recognize that others may tolerate forms of real dairy balanced amongst other real food groups. The Sephardic culture is entrenched in many forms of dairy foods. Back in the days in the old country, their dairy products were fresh and real, milked from cows that were grass-fed. Here are some of the staple foods that are a mainstay in the Syrian market:

CHEESE

The unique cheese flavor is rich and salty. It is a staple at meals, especially at a brunch-type setting, and also comes in a form to be strung, aka "string cheese," with the added flavor of a seed from the nigella sativa plant that looks like a black seed and tastes like pepper.

YOGURT

Syrians make a specialty yogurt called Laban. It is a cultured kefir-like dairy product, rich in natural probiotics, that has a sour flavor resembling that of plain Greek yogurt. A patient of mine born in Lebanon loves to eat a dish that combines the Laban with olive oil and zaatar spice for a creamy spread on foods like pita bread.

It is easy to get lost in the debate over dairy. The reality is that our food industry has leaps and bounds to take before it can be a trusted real-food source. It is far from perfect, so it is difficult to make our real-food, real-life goals about perfection. Instead, make an educated decision by weighing the benefits and risks of adding different foods to your diet. Then, see if there are other foods that provide the same benefits with less risk and try incorporating them more in your real-food diet. Eating the right forms of dairy, in moderation, can be tolerable and healthful in

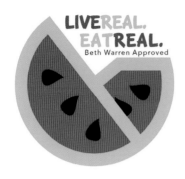

your real life. It also fits into Steps Two and Three of my Steps to Living a Real Life with Real Food, as meat and dairy are both protein sources that can be incorporated as one-fourth of your plate for meals and as part of your real-food snacks. Be sure to keep in mind Step 1 and eat no less than two hours and no more than four hours apart if you are eating dairy first. Following the kashrut laws, if you ate meat first, you need to wait six hours before you can consume dairy. Check out the meal plans for ways to balance both meat and dairy foods in context of a real-food diet so you do not overdo each one.

I enjoy eating cultured dairy products like yogurt and kefir. Beneficial bacteria and lactic acid are produced in prominent Middle Eastern fermented milk and cheese products, like Lebne, and are proven to have the ability to kill pathogens as well as modulate the immune system.[72] I also find that many people suffering from intolerance may tolerate cultured dairy because they contain probiotics and enzymes to help digest the sugars in the dairy. Additionally, cottage cheese has more protein and less lactose and is considered a lean meat in the food-exchange list. These quality sources of protein are considered helpful in our path toward better health.

The research from either side of the cow's milk debate shows that, in small quantities, it is not harmful. The issue I find with milk and dairy is the same for the other controversial food groups. People may consume too much dairy or too much cow's milk. The amount increases the dairy sensitivity threshold and leads to intolerances. When you lower that threshold, the tolerance for a small amount, balanced amongst other whole food groups, helps with better digestion. Then you can bask in the benefits of dairy (consumed in moderation), including its high protein content, calcium, and vitamins A and D without the intolerable side effects.

Milk is one product that I buy organic for the same reason I support grass-fed meat: it is safer to consume since the entire makeup of the cow and, therefore, the milk quality, is different. I am comfortable with drinking a small amount of whole milk, in my coffee for example, because it has the positive health benefits of natural CLA and is less processed.

Overall, I limit my cow's milk intake and substitute with non-dairy sources of milk, like almond and coconut. It is better to rotate your food choices and keep your body "guessing" on what new foods it will have. Like a little boy who runs to his mother to open a new gift, he eagerly shreds the wrapping paper, exclaims "Wow!" with excitement over the new truck, and spends the next hour figuring out new ways to use the toy, even though he has four other trucks sitting in the toy closet. The old ones lost their excitement and freshness, but the new one changed the child in that moment, just like new foods will change up your metabolism.

Keep in mind that dairy tolerance depends on a healthy gut. If you are experiencing flatulence, bloating, or more severe symptoms mentioned, I would recommend keeping dairy out of your diet. If you don't, you may increase inflammation in the gut and body, a chronic state we are looking to avoid by eating real foods.

In the end, despite what any marketing makes you think, cow's milk is not a vital food group, but rather a food *product*. If you are concerned or uncomfortable with consuming dairy, there are many alternatives to cow's milk to get your calcium and other vitamin and mineral needs. As a result, cow's milk is not essential, but it *is* an easier option . . . and easy is not necessarily healthier.

Here are ways to increase your calcium intake from non-dairy sources in your cooking (see Recipes):

1. Add tofu to your meals, such as stir-frying with vegetables.
2. Leafy greens, like kale, are an added source of calcium, so try steaming them or add them to casseroles, soups, and stews.

3. Non-dairy sources of milk, such as almond milk, contains calcium. Use them in recipes such as pancakes, pudding, and oatmeal (see Recipes).
4. Stir a drizzle of blackstrap molasses into your oatmeal.
5. Almond butter is higher in calcium than peanut butter, so rotate the natural nut butters.
6. Try adding beans, like black-eyed peas, to soups and salads.

ALTERNATIVE MILK SOURCES

Goat's Milk

Interestingly, the most cited source for the kashrut laws against mixing milk with meat reference states "[a] kid 'goat' in his mother's milk"—it doesn't say a word about cows! Although it is dairy-based, goat's milk closely mimics the breast milk of humans.[73] As a result, someone intolerant to cow's milk may tolerate goat's milk because it is easier to digest.

The allergic reaction to cow's milk is largely due to the high levels of the protein Alpha S1 Casein. In goat's milk, those levels are 89 percent less and are different in structure, resulting in a less-allergenic food.[74] Researchers in one study fed dairy-allergic infants goat's milk and 93 percent experienced virtually no side effects.[75]

Furthermore, goat's milk differs from cow's milk in its homogenization. Goat's milk undergoes natural homogenization (the process of allowing the milk and cream components to stay combined upon standing); whereas cow's milk requires a processed homogenization.

Nutritionally, goat's milk has a greater amount of essential fatty acids than cow's milk; it also has significantly greater amounts of copper, manganese, vitamin B6, vitamin A and D, niacin, and potassium and 15 percent more calcium.[76] It is also a good source of phosphorous and riboflavin (vitamin B2).

Goat's milk, per cup: 168 calories, 10g of fat (7g saturated fat), 11g sugars, 0g fiber, 9g protein

Hemp Milk

Hemp milk is an excellent source of Omega-3 fats, providing your daily requirement in a single serving—that's four times as much as soy milk and six times as much as cow's milk. The downside is its lower protein content than the other forms of milk.

A few studies show that hemp seeds may improve the function of our immune system, promote healthy skin and hair, and boost cognitive performance.[77]

You can also use hemp seeds for a protein and Omega-3 boost. Add to smoothies, soups, yogurt, and other liquid-based foods.

Hemp Milk, per cup: 70 calories, 6g fat (0.5 g saturated), 0g sugars, 0g fiber, 2–4g protein
Taste: Grain-like and nutty

Almond Milk

If you want a low-calorie and low-sugar option, almond milk is a better choice compared to other non-dairy milks, but it's also lower in protein. Almond milk is a good source of heart-healthy monounsaturated fats, natural calcium, magnesium, manganese, selenium, and Vitamin E. Vitamin E and selenium act as antioxidants that protect the cell membranes, improve our immune system, and aid in reproduction and thyroid function.[78]

Almond Milk, per cup: 45 calories, 3.5g fat (0 g saturated), 0g sugars, 1g fiber, 2g protein
Taste: A slightly sweet almond flavor

Oat Milk

Oat milk is a unique non-dairy source because it offers both fiber and a moderate amount of protein. On the flip side, it has more sugar than the other options, is cholesterol and lactose free, and also has high levels of antioxidant vitamin E. It also contains folic acid, which is needed to synthesize and repair DNA, produce healthy red blood cells, and prevent anemia.

Unfortunately, oat milk is considerably more processed due to the addition of the ingredients carrageenan and vitamin A palmitate.

> **Oat Milk**, per cup: 130 calories, 2.5g fat (0 g saturated), 19g sugars, 2g fiber, 4g protein
> Taste: Oatmeal-like taste and mildly sweet with a watery consistency

If you're worried about an allergic reaction, rice milk is your best bet, as it is known to be a non-allergenic food. However, it is also the lowest in protein and may be higher in sugar and calories. Some people also report constipation.

The beneficial unsaturated fat is derived from rice bran oil, which can help lower your blood cholesterol. The vitamins niacin and B6 also aid in cholesterol control, while the high magnesium content helps to control your blood pressure. Iron and copper in rice milk increase your red blood cell production, giving you more vitality as a result of better oxygenated blood.

> **Rice Milk**, per cup: 120 calories, 2.5g fat (0 g saturated), 10g sugars, 0g fiber, 1g protein
> Taste: Oatmeal-like taste and mildly sweet with a watery consistency

Soy Milk

Soy milk is the most comparable to cow's milk in protein: 8–11 grams per cup—but can be higher in sugar. Soy milk has traces of fiber and is derived solely from plant sources.

However, there is debate over soy products (see chapter 8). It is important to note that the soy protein looks similar to dairy and is also one of the seven main food allergens (wheat, soy, dairy, fish, shellfish, peanuts, and tree nuts). If you are suspicious of a dairy intolerance, you should eliminate soy in the diet, as well, and then add it back in later to test for tolerance.

Unfortunately, soy milk does not contain natural calcium or vitamin B12, although some products are fortified with them. See chapter 9 for the debate over the benefits and risks of soy products.

> **Soy Milk**, per cup, unsweetened: 80 calories, 4.3g fat (0.5 g saturated fat), 1g sugar, 1.5g fiber, 7g protein
> Taste: Chalky tasting in the plain variety but if sweetened with flavors like vanilla and chocolate to mask the taste, it adds a lot of sugar

Coconut Milk

Coconut milk is a great dairy-free alternative for those who are lactose intolerant, allergic to animal milk, or want to substitute for milk or cream in baking to make the food "pareve." Although all five grams of fat in coconut milk are saturated, these fats are medium-chain fatty acids and are metabolized differently than the long-chain fats associated with animal meat and atherosclerosis (see chapter 4). Medium-chain fatty acids are sent directly to the liver, where they are used and burned immediately as energy. They may increase metabolism, slow digestion, improve the immune system, and boost cognitive development (see chapter 4).

Coconut milk is also rich in lauric acid, which is also found in human milk and is shown to have anti-viral and anti-bacterial properties. Unlike other nut or plant milks, the saturated fat content of coconut milk is significant at 5 grams per serving, is also lower in protein and calcium, and may have added preservatives like vitamin A palmitate and carrageenan, so rotate this dairy-free alternative amongst other lower-calorie options like almond milk.

Coconut Milk, per cup: 50 calories, 5g fat (5 g saturated), 0g sugars, 0g fiber, 1g protein
Taste: Creamy and thick texture with a rich flavor

CALCIUM-RICH FOOD

Dairy Food	Amount	Calcium in mg
Milk	1 cup	300
Yogurt	1 cup	275
Sour cream	1 cup	265
Cheddar cheese	30 gm	200
Cottage cheese	1 cup	155
Feta cheese	30 gm	140
Ice cream	1/2 cup	85
Non-Dairy Food		
Molasses	2 tablespoons	340
Canned sardines	100 gm	325
White beans	1 cup	190
Arugula (gargeer)	1 cup	150
Almonds, Walnuts, Hazelnuts and Sunflower seeds	¼ cup	140
Tahina	2 tablespoons	130
Oranges	2 medium	100
Broccoli	1 cup	95
Chickpeas	1 cup	80
Whole grain cereal (calcium fortified)	3/4 cup	1000
Cooked spinach	1 cup	450

CALCIUM NEEDS

AGE	AMOUNT OF DAILY CALCIUM
6 months - 1 year *	600 mg
1 – 10 years	800 – 1200 mg
11 – 24 years	1200 – 1500 mg
Adult Women	
Pregnant or nursing	1200 – 1500 mg
25 – 49 years (pre-menopausal)	1000 mg
Over 50 years	1500 mg
Adult Men	
25 – 64 years	1000 mg
Over 65 years	1500 mg

CHAPTER 6

GRAINS AND THE REAL-FOOD DIET

"If there is no flour, there is no Torah."
—*Pirkei Avot 3:21*

During ancient times, the Israelites lived a predominately rural life. As a result, many of the laws and lifestyle references in the Bible were about agricultural methods.

The first reference to grains was after the fall of man from the Garden of Eden. G–d told Adam that man will, "[t]ill the soil until death . . . From the sweat of your brow shall you get bread to eat, until you return to the ground from which you were taken." As man's punishment after the first sin of eating the fruits from the Tree of Life, he had to harvest the field in order to eat bread. Grains were referenced with Adam's sons shortly after. Cain dedicated a grain offering to G–d, but G–d preferred an animal offering made by his brother, Abel.

The Bible continued to refer to grains in times of hardship. When the Israelites went on their Exodus out of Egypt, they only had enough time to make unleavened bread. Earlier, during the seven years of famine in Egypt, Joseph could only store grains and that was all the people had to eat. Later, during Ezekiel's reign, there are many references to grains. G–d commanded him to carefully portion and use "[w]heat and barley, and beans and lentils, and millet and spelt" to make a bread for the people to eat. Ezekiel protested eating them and argued they are a food for animals. Should we feel as negative about incorporating grains into our diets as these depressing biblical references?

Gluten, the protein in wheat, and other characteristics of grains are swept up in controversy. The gluten-free fad diet is rampant. About eighteen million Americans have some degree of gluten sensitivity.[79, 80] As a result, the sale and introduction of gluten-free products are thriving at a rapid pace. Spins, a market-research-and-consulting firm for the natural-products industry, reported that sales of gluten-free food grew 27 percent between 2009 and 2011—from $4.8 billion in 2009 to $5.4 billion in 2010 to an estimated $6.1 billion in 2011. Companies like Amy's® Kitchen, Bob's Red Mill®, and Udi's® Gluten Free Foods, which have some kosher-certified products, are reporting huge growth.

Even Kellogg's® introduced gluten-free Rice Krispies® in 2011 and other companies like Frito-Lay® and Post® Foods were not far behind in stamping their gluten-free seal, which identifies less than 20 parts-per-million gluten on some products. The company, ConAgra Mills®, a leading flour supplier, published a report characterizing gluten-free specialty products as a $486 million industry.[81]

With all the obvious hype, should we jump on the gluten-free bandwagon, or is it only for the handful of intolerant? What is the bigger picture of the function of grains inside our bodies?

In this chapter, I will show you how grains can fit into your real-food diet.

GRAINS: HARVESTING THE TRUTH

Medical conditions including celiac disease, gluten intolerance, type II diabetes, heart disease, and cancer are real problems in the United States and around the world. They have a common link: chronic inflammation.[82] Chronic inflammation also causes an altered metabolism, higher adiposity, and impaired insulin sensitivity, which gives a strong link to overweight and obesity.

Some studies link grains to inflammation, arterial plaque, joint problems, rheumatoid arthritis, infertility, and PCOS symptoms.[83] Celiac disease is shown to be a more common but neglected disorder than has generally been recognized in the United States. Yet, non-celiac gluten sensitivity (NCGS) is increasingly shown to be a larger issue, as well. In a double-blind, randomized, placebo-controlled rechallenge, researchers found that patients with IBS but without celiac disease[84] experienced alleviation of symptoms following a gluten-free diet. Previous researchers reported that approximately 20 percent of patients (24 out of 120 subjects) with IBS experienced food sensitivities and found relief when eliminating wheat and dairy from their diets.[85]

I have witnessed different effects of grains with my patients. Here are the two sides of the debate:

Going With or Against the Grain

Some circles, such as the paleo-diet followers, argue that the chemical components gluten, lectin, and phytates can be harmful for our health if they are not neutralized. Phytates, they claim, may interfere with the absorption of calcium, zinc, magnesium, copper, and iron,[86]—some of the very nutrients we want to absorb through our grain consumption.

Interestingly, the same phytates the anti-grain movement cautions against, the pro-grain group advocates as having some health benefits, including anti-inflammatory effects. Research shows phytates help to normalize cell growth and stop the proliferation of cancer cells. They also may help prevent cardiovascular disease and lower the glycemic load of a food.[87]

In the end, there is does not appear to be any substantial evidence to support the significance of any harmful affects of phytates in humans. Incorporating a real life with other real foods promotes a balance of all food groups, which will offset any inhibitory affects of certain vitamins and minerals within grains, if they may exist.

FERMENTED GRAINS

Interestingly, the Israelites seemed to enjoy a healthier consumption of grains during biblical times. They prepared grains by soaking, fermenting, or sprouting them before eating. The process may have not been intentional, but because of environmentally warm and moist storage conditions, sprouting and fermentation likely occurred. During the ritual Seder on the Passover holiday, we read that the Israelites ate unleavened bread because it did not "[h]ave time to ferment," which seemed to be normal protocol.

The process of sprouting grains changes the structure of those potentially harmful chemical components and reduces their effects. Fermentation further improves the composition of some minerals in grains.[88] A lot of issues people have with grains can be alleviated with proper preparation techniques.

What can be sprouted?

Grains	Sunflower seeds
Alfalfa	Lentils
Clover	Mung beans
Broccoli	Wheat berries
Radish	Chickpeas

The brand, Food for Life® by Ezekiel 4:9® products, are made from sprouted grain products.

In addition, grains of my ancestors were often ground by hand using stones or similar objects. The size of the hand-ground, sprouted grain was a lot larger than the powdered flour of today. Because of the increase in surface area from the flour, the starch composition expanded. All carbohydrates break down to sugar in the body, yet our starchy flour converts more quickly into sugar in the blood than the ground grains of biblical times. Therefore, the glycemic index of more refined flour particles is higher than the flour with larger particles, which does not help our health.

Additionally, the most processed form of grain detailed in the Bible was bread, as opposed to all the starch-filled processed products of today: cookies, cakes, and crackers, combined with other processed ingredients and preservatives that would be equivalent to my ancestors reading a foreign language. It seems the manifestation of what starch has become in our diets—overeaten, heavily processed foods, refined grains with tons of unrecognizable and manmade ingredients—is what is hurting us.

STARCHES AND THE REAL LIFE WITH REAL FOOD DIET

You will be happy to hear that my real-food diet with whole grains promotes anti-inflammatory ways, which can help build a strong resistance against diabetes, cancer, and heart disease, making a healthier you! It is important to rotate your carbohydrate sources from grains to quality starchy vegetables like beets, sweet potatoes, potatoes, and beans (see chapter 7 and chapter 8). Remember Step Two of Steps to Living a Real Life with Real Food: starches should account for only one-quarter of your nine-inch plate (see Serving Size of Starch). If you notice through your food diary that your "go-to" starch source is bread, for example, change it up! Oftentimes, inflammation is promoted not by grains alone, but by the repetition of the source of grain you are eating. Choosing quality whole grains, and preparing them in a "biblical fashion" if needed, can help you best tolerate this vital food group.

Serving of Starch Options

½ cup cooked rice, bulgur, pasta, or cooked cereal

1 ounce dry pasta, rice, or other dry grain

1 slice bread

1 small muffin (weighing 1 ounce)

1 cup ready-to-eat cereal flakes

WHOLESOME WHOLE GRAINS [89]

Consumption of whole grains is widely favored over refined grains. Whole grains contain their entire composition intact: the germ, endosperm, and bran.

WHAT IS IN A WHOLE GRAIN?

Because of their whole form, whole grains are naturally high in fiber, protein, B vitamins, and the minerals iron, magnesium, phosphorous, zinc, manganese, copper, and selenium.

Iron

Iron helps our bodies make hemoglobin (for red blood cells) and myoglobin (for muscles), both of which help carry and store oxygen. Iron also plays a role in many other routine bodily functions.

Magnesium

Magnesium is an essential mineral required for hundreds of biochemical reactions, including transmission of nerve impulses, converting food into energy, body temperature regulation, and maintaining a strong immune system. It also helps us absorb calcium for healthy bones and teeth.

Phosphorus

Another essential mineral, phosphorus is present in every cell in your body, making up 1 percent of your body weight. Its main function is the formation of bones and teeth, but it's also the key to the synthesis of protein for cell repair, growth, and maintenance; for heartbeat regularity; and for nerve conduction.

Zinc

The mineral zinc helps your immune system fight off bacteria and viruses and helps wounds heal. It also helps your body make proteins and DNA. Zinc is also essential to proper functioning of your sense of taste and smell.

Copper

Copper (another mineral) helps us absorb iron and also helps regulate blood pressure and heart rate. Copper is also needed for the production of melanin, which colors our hair and skin.

Manganese

The mineral manganese helps us handle oxidative stress. It activates many important enzymes in the body that are crucial to metabolism of carbohydrates, amino acids, and cholesterol. Manganese is also essential to the formation of healthy cartilage and bone.

Selenium

Selenium is a trace mineral. Although we only need small amounts of it, it is essential to helping prevent cellular damage from free radicals, to regulating thyroid function, and for a healthy immune system.

B Vitamins

The many B vitamins help with metabolism, the process your body uses to make energy from the food you eat. While each has its own functions, in general they also help maintain healthy skin, hair, and muscles; form red blood cells; and promote healthy immune and nervous system function. Some research shows that B vitamins also prevent mood swings.

Source: www.wholegrainscouncil.org

MORE ON FIBER

I favor whole grain consumption largely due to the naturally high fiber content. Fiber deserves a chapter all to itself. It is a superhero nutrient shown to reduce blood pressure, lower low-density lipoprotein (LDL) and cholesterol levels (see chapter 4), and ease inflammation. It can also increase the weight and size of your stool and prevent hemorrhoids.

Dietary fiber is a component of carbohydrates. It includes both insoluble and soluble forms. Both types of fiber are equally important for digestion and preventing conditions such as heart disease, diabetes, obesity, diverticulitis, and constipation.[90]

Insoluble Fiber

Because this type of fiber does not dissolve in water, it is responsible for improving your digestive system. Insoluble fiber promotes gut health by acting as a natural laxative and adds bulk to the diet, alleviating constipation.

Sources of Insoluble Fiber: Whole wheat, whole grains, wheat bran, corn bran, seeds, nuts, barley, couscous, brown rice, bulgur, zucchini, celery, broccoli, cabbage, onions, tomatoes, carrots, cucumbers, green beans, dark leafy vegetables, raisins, grapes, fruit, and root vegetable skins.

Soluble Fiber

Soluble fiber has the opposite affect as insoluble fiber because it absorbs water. It forms a gel inside the gut and slows digestion, which aids in weight control. The affects of soluble fiber allow you to feel fuller for longer by slowing gastric emptying time. Foods high in soluble fiber have a lower glycemic index, which poses another positive effect on insulin sensitivity—it lowers the risk for diabetes. It is also good for LDL cholesterol (see chapter 4), since the bulk and gel-like consistency draws cholesterol from the gut and interferes with its absorption.

Sources of Soluble Fiber: oatmeal, oat cereal, lentils, apples, oranges, pears, oat bran, strawberries, nuts, flaxseeds, beans, dried peas, blueberries, psyllium, cucumbers, celery, and carrots.

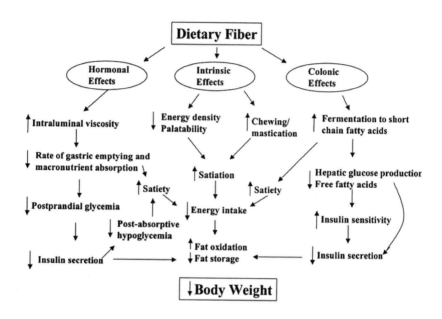

Source: Pereira and Ludwig

I stamp my Kosher Seal of Approval on consuming fiber-filled foods to feel full at and in between meals and snacks. Ideally, the options should be from real-food sources (see Meal Plans), as opposed to foods fortified with fiber.

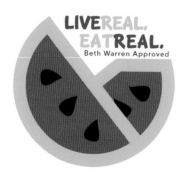

The process of fortification adds a nutrient into a food that does not naturally occur. Enhancing the fiber content in Fruit Loops® and Apple Jacks® in 2009, for example, did not make these cereals a healthier food. Always look at a product as a whole and what it is doing for your health, and then make your choice.

Most Americans get only about 15 grams of fiber per day in their diets. But the 2005 Dietary Guidelines for Americans recommends about 25 grams for women under fifty and teenage girls. Teenage boys and men under fifty (who consume more calories than women) require as much as 30 to 38 grams of dietary fiber daily.

When you begin adding more fiber into your diet, do not be worried if you experience symptoms of bloating and flatulence. Drink more water to offset these side effects. As you incorporate consistently more fiber, your body will adjust to the intake and you will reap the fiber benefits of increased fullness, a flatter belly, and improved digestion.

MORE ON WHOLE GRAINS

When I recommended that Shirley, a patient, consume only whole grains and no refined grains, I was met with a look of disgust: "Ew, I hate those whole-wheat noodles and there is no way I am eating brown rice." Because white rice is a staple to many of my Syrian meals and often combined with other dishes, I am not surprised by the reluctance. However, I often find a patient's limited knowledge of whole grains goes as far as whole wheat and brown rice. In fact, there are many other whole grains to choose from. I fully encourage you to view the more extensive list on wholegrainscouncil.org, but here is a glimpse of the most common ones I encounter in patients' diets and my own cuisine. Try different forms, brands, and ways of preparation and, most importantly, do not give up! (See Recipes.)

TYPES OF WHOLE GRAINS

o **Amaranth**

Today amaranth is becoming more popular, thanks to a lively, peppery taste and a higher level of protein (roughly 13–14 percent protein) compared to most other grains. I have one patient who tolerates only amaranth with her IBS symptoms and cannot go one morning without making it just like hot oatmeal.

It can also be popped like corn. Amaranth doesn't have gluten, so it must be mixed with wheat to make leavened breads. It is popular in cereals, breads, muffins, crackers, and pancakes.

- *Health bonus:* Amaranth's complete protein contains lysine, an amino acid missing or negligible in many grains.

o **Barley**

Barley is one of the oldest cultivated grains and is referenced multiple times in the Bible. Hulled barley, available at health-food stores, retains more whole-grain nutrients, but cooks slowly. Lightly pearled barley is not technically a whole grain (as small amounts of the bran are missing)—but it is full of fiber and much healthier than a fully-refined grain.

- *Health bonus:* The fiber in barley is especially healthy; it may lower cholesterol even more effectively than oat fiber. The beta-glucan in barley is a form of fiber that improves insulin resistance. It also has tocopherols and tocotrienols, otherwise known as vitamin E.

o **Brown rice**

Whole-grain rice is usually brown—but, unknown to many, can also be black, purple, red, or any of a variety of exotic hues. Brown rice is lower in fiber than most other whole grains, but rich in many nutrients.

- *Health bonus:* Rice is one of the most easily-digested grains—one reason rice cereal is often recommended as a baby's first solid. This makes rice ideal for those on a restricted diet or who are gluten-intolerant.

o **Buckwheat**

Buckwheat goes way beyond the pancake mixes we associate with it (although I do love Bob's Red Mill® buckwheat pancake mix!). Botanically, buckwheat is a cousin of rhubarb, not technically a grain at all—and certainly not a kind of wheat. But its nutrients, nutty flavor, and appearance have led to its ready adoption into the family of grains. Buckwheat tolerates poor soil, grows well on rocky hillsides, and thrives without chemical pesticides.

- *Health bonus:* Buckwheat is the only grain known to have high levels of an antioxidant called rutin, which studies show improves circulation and prevents LDL cholesterol from blocking blood vessels.

o **Bulgur (cracked wheat)**

When wheat kernels are boiled, dried, cracked, and then sorted by size, the result is bulgur. This wheat product is sometimes referred to as Middle Eastern pasta for its versatility as a base for all sorts of dishes. Bulgur is most often made from durum wheat, but in fact almost any wheat—hard or soft, red or white—can be made into bulgur. Because bulgur has been precooked and dried, it needs to be boiled for only about ten minutes to be ready to eat—about the same time as dry pasta. This makes bulgur an extremely nutritious fast food for quick side dishes, pilafs, or salads. Perhaps bulgur's best-known traditional use is the salad bazargan (see Recipes). Cracked wheat cooks faster, as the wheat berries have been split open, allowing water to penetrate more quickly. Some stores also sell wheat flakes, which look similar to rolled oats.

- *Health bonus:* Bulgur has more fiber than quinoa, oats, millet, buckwheat, or corn. Its quick cooking time and mild flavor make it ideal for those new to whole-grain cooking.

o **Whole-wheat pasta or couscous**

Wheat (Exodus 29:2) and barley (Kings 4:42) were shown to be the primary components of bread during the biblical days. Wheat was preferred, but it was also more expensive than barley and less available in hard times.

Wheat has come to dominate the grains we eat because it contains large amounts of gluten, a stretchy protein that enables bakers to create satisfying risen breads. Two main varieties of wheat are widely eaten. *Durum wheat* is made into pasta, while bread wheat is used for most other wheat foods. *Hard wheat*, a type of bread wheat, has more protein, including more gluten, and is used for bread, while *soft wheat* creates "cake flour" with lower protein. Like the other grains above, wheat can be enjoyed in many different forms in addition to baked goods and pasta.

When you are shopping for wheat, look for the term *whole wheat* to make sure you are getting all the bran, germ, and endosperm. Just plain wheat legally refers to refined wheat.

o **Oats**

Oats have a sweet flavor that makes them a favorite for breakfast cereals. Unique among grains, oats almost never have their bran and germ removed during processing. So if you see oats or oat flour on the label, relax: you are virtually guaranteed to be getting whole grain.

In the United States, most oats are steamed and flattened to produce "old-fashioned" or regular oats, quick oats, and instant oats. The more that oats are flattened and steamed, the quicker they cook and the softer they become. If you prefer a chewier, nuttier texture, consider steel-cut oats, also sometimes called Irish or Scottish oats. Steel-cut oats consist of the entire oat kernel (similar in look to a grain of rice), sliced once or twice into smaller pieces to help water penetrate and cook the grain. Cooked for about twenty minutes, steel-cut oats create a breakfast porridge that delights many people who think they do not love oatmeal!

- *Health bonus:* Scientific studies have concluded that, like barley, oats contain a special kind of fiber called beta-glucan, which is found to be especially effective in lowering cholesterol. Recent research reports indicate that oats also have a unique antioxidant, avenanthramides, which help protect blood vessels from the damaging effects of LDL cholesterol. They are also very high in tryptophan and selenium, which affect mood.

o **Quinoa**

Quinoa (keen-wah) is botanically a relative of Swiss chard and beets rather than a "true" grain. It cooks in about 10 to 12 minutes, creating a light, fluffy side dish. Quinoa can also be incorporated into soups, salads, and baked goods. Commercially, quinoa is now appearing in cereal flakes and other processed foods.

Quinoa is a small, light-colored, round grain, similar in appearance to sesame seeds. But quinoa is also available in other colors, including red, purple, and black. Most quinoa must be rinsed before cooking to remove the bitter residue of saponins, a plant-defense that wards off insects.

- *Health bonus:* The abundant protein in quinoa is complete protein, which means it contains all the essential amino acids our bodies can't make on their own. It is also high in potassium, which helps give us flatter bellies!

o **Rye**

Rye is unusual among grains for the high level of fiber in its endosperm—not just in its bran. Because of this, rye products generally have a lower glycemic index than products made from wheat and most other grains, making them especially healthy for diabetics.

Be sure to look for whole rye or rye berries in the ingredient list—just because something is labeled "rye bread" doesn't guarantee it's whole grain.

o **Spelt**

Spelt can be used in place of common wheat in most recipes. Like other varieties of wheat, spelt can be found in both whole and refined form in our food supply—so look for the words *whole spelt.*

- *Health bonus:* Spelt is higher in protein than common wheat. There are anecdotal reports that some people sensitive to wheat can tolerate spelt, but no reliable medical studies have addressed that issue.

o **Wheat berries**

Wheat berries—whole-wheat kernels—can also be cooked as a side dish or breakfast cereal, but must be boiled for about an hour, preferably after soaking overnight. Moroccans use wheat berries in a different version of Chamin, a stew-like dish traditionally eaten on the Sabbath (see Recipe).

o **Wild rice**

Wild rice is not technically rice at all, but the seed of an aquatic grass. The strong flavor and high price of wild rice means that it is most often consumed in a blend with other rice varieties or other grains. Wild rice has twice the protein and fiber of brown rice, but less iron and calcium.

o **Other grains include**

Triticale, Kamut® (which has higher levels of protein than common wheat and more Vitamin E), Sorghum (a gluten-free grain popular amongst those with celiac disease), Teff (which has over twice the iron compared with other grains and three times the calcium), and Millet.

STARCHY VEGETABLES

Although vegetables are essential in our diets, some are considered "starchy" and account for about 15 grams of carbs, 3 grams of protein, and about 80 calories. To fulfill Steps Two and Three of my Steps to Living a Real Life with Real Food, these starchy vegetables, along with whole grains, should be reserved for the one-quarter portion of starches on your plate and as the "fiber" of your protein and fiber real-food snack:

o   Beans (Beans can also account for the protein portion of your snack. See chapter 8.)
o   Beets
o   Carrots
o   Corn
o   Green Peas
o   Parsnips
o   Plantain
o   Pumpkin
o   Sweet Potatoes
o   White Potatoes
o   Winter Squash, such as acorn or butternut squash
o   Yams

Tips on How to Incorporate Whole Grains into Your Real-Food Diet

o   Read labels. Look for the word *whole* before any grains on the ingredient list and check the number of grams of dietary fiber on the nutrition facts panel of packages to select high-fiber foods.
o   Start your day with a high-fiber cereal that contains at least 5 grams of fiber per serving.
o   Snack on raw vegetables and fruits in combination with a protein.
o   Add legumes, seeds, and nuts into soups, salads, and stews.

Replace refined white bread, pasta, and rice with 100 percent whole-grain products.

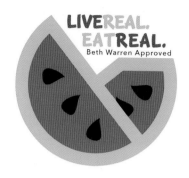

I stamp my Kosher Seal of Approval on whole grains, eaten in moderation, balanced with other vital food groups for better health. Whole grains have nutrients we need such as, iron, potassium, magnesium, fiber, and B vitamins.

If there is an issue with grain consumption, it is that people develop a "carb-centric" diet. Carbohydrates break down into sugar and research has shown that sugar becomes an addiction like one to cocaine. It causes a euphoric effect that triggers dopamine, the chemical that controls pleasure in the brain.[91] As a result, your threshold of fulfilling a carbohydrate craving increases over time until the majority of your food intake becomes carbs! Sugar craves more sugar.

The problem lies not in the consumption of quality whole grains, but the proportion of whole grains in context of other food groups. Studies show consuming a low refined carbohydrate, high-fiber diet will help you lose and maintain weight and add to your overall health by improving conditions such as non-alcoholic fatty liver, metabolic syndrome, and obesity.[92]

During a patient's food recall, I aim to identify his or her food preferences and uncover one food group as responsible for the majority intake. Almost always, that means carbohydrates, by a description of a potato-chip, bread-loving diet. The goal of that patient's medical nutrition therapy is to incorporate quality foods like healthy fats, fruits, and vegetables into the diet to lower the threshold of carbohydrate sensitivity and achieve a real-food balance. While you are filling out your food diaries (see Food and Mood Diary), it is important to recognize a "carb-centric" trend to your food preferences.

I began to refer to carbohydrates as "a fiber" to my patients. Because of the cringe I see when I recommend they eat "a carb," I found it safer to refer to them as a fiber-food because a fruit or a piece of bread will fulfill an intake of carbohydrate or eventual glucose for energy. After all, carbohydrates are made of fiber and sugars, so whether it is a piece of bread or an apple, anything can fit into a real-food diet as long as the products in question are whole grains or fresh fruits, both rotated and balanced.

The important part to remember is that although whole grain carbohydrates can be a part of all meals and snacks (including fruits), you should never aim to get *full* on carbs. If you are technically able to eat two slices of bread with lunch, but are full and satisfied with one, then stop. The longer you live a real life with real food, the more you will trust your belly to tell you when you've had enough starch. You also should not eat the starch portion first. If you take a bite of pasta, chances are that you'll finish eating it quickly and, without thinking, go for more pasta and overconsume carbs.

Carbohydrate foods should be a side dish amongst the larger portion of vegetables and some lean protein consumed with meals (refer to Step Two of my Steps to Living a Real Life with Real Food) or combined with protein to fulfill Step 3. With that in mind, it is safe to consume foods with carbs at all meals and snacks to achieve weight loss and better health.

For the other patients I have seen with sincere gluten intolerance, celiac disease, IBS, and other food allergies and sensitivities related to grains, it is clear they do not tolerate gluten. Their symptoms may be accompanied by an increase in blood levels of the antibody to gluten. Other people who do not experience any signs in their bloodwork may have non-celiac gluten sensitivity (NCGS). The majority of symptoms associated with NCGS are subjective, including abdominal pain, headache, "brain fog," tingling and/or numbness in hands and feet, fatigue, and musculoskeletal pain.[93]

Researchers in Australia showed that participants with IBS who did not also have celiac disease, found they were able to control their symptoms under a gluten-free diet.[94] Each person was asked to eat two slices of bread and one muffin daily, one group of participants ate foods with gluten, while there was no gluten in the food consumed by the placebo group. Nine participants of the gluten group stopped the study diet prematurely because of intolerable symptoms. During the entire study period, scores for pain, stool consistency, and tiredness were significantly worse in the gluten group than in the placebo group.

The study provides some of the most convincing evidence for the existence of non-celiac gluten intolerance. The study concluded by reminding of the "[n]ecessity of strict, lifelong adherence to a gluten-free diet; an increased cancer risk if exposed to gluten; and the need to screen family members."[95]

If you suspect a non-celiac gluten sensitivity, try an elimination diet under the care of a qualified registered dietitian to identify which types of grains are intolerable. Slowly, reintroduce grains and gauge your gluten tolerance threshold. Symptoms of an intolerance can include stomach pains, bloat, heartburn, joint pains, headache, skin rashes, fatigue, insomnia, and brain fog. It is best to get tested for celiac disease before attempting a gluten-free diet so you can have a more accurate result.

Real Life, Real Food, Real Story

One of my patients, Sandra, developed late onset celiac disease in her twenties. As a result of misdiagnosis, she had severe inflammation and decreased gut integrity. As a result, she was not absorbing components of her food, especially starches, which caused other problems throughout her body.

Multiple-sugar bonds, like disaccharides and polysaccharides, need to break down in the gut with the release of essential enzymes and other components. The process relies on a healthy gut. If you have impaired gut integrity, there are many foods you cannot tolerate. As we worked to bolster her gut by eliminating all sources of gluten and including other fermented, cultured foods, probiotics, and a lot of veggies and fruits, we reintroduced gluten-free grains. Because of her sensitive state, she sprouted all her grains, trying foods like brown rice and quinoa in miniscule amounts (sometimes a tablespoon at a time), to ease the digestive process in her gut and build a tolerance for these foods. In similar situations, with chronic inflammation and decreased gut integrity, I recommend beginning to incorporate grains (preferably sprouted) slowly, since the enzymes are intact and your gut does not have to do as much work to break down the starches and absorb the food. The goal is to work up to optimal tolerance without exacerbating inflammation or other symptoms.

For the majority of us with healthy guts and no other applicable medical conditions, we can incorporate small quantities of whole grains into our diets, allowing our bodies to handle the peaks in blood sugar and insulin, our sugar cravings to be kept at bay in the healthiest way, and our bodies to take advantage of the vitamins, minerals, and preferred source of energy—the carbohydrates—they provide.

CHAPTER 7

FRUITS AND VEGETABLES—HOW TO CHOOSE GOOD PRODUCE

*"Vegetables provide a nutritious and inexpensive addition
allowing a scholar to subsist on a smaller income and devote
time to Torah study."*

—Rashi, commentating on the Talmud, 140b

*[2] And the woman said unto the serpent, We may eat of the fruit
of the trees of the garden:[3] But of the fruit of the tree which is
in the midst of the garden, G–d has said, You shall not eat of it,
neither shall you touch it, lest you die*

*⁷ And the eyes of them both were opened, and they [Adam
and Eve] knew that they were naked; and they sewed fig
leaves together, and made themselves aprons.*

—Gen. 3:2–7

Fruits and vegetables have the most positive and consistent research backing their consumption amongst all food groups. A school of thought does not exist that forbids its consumption. Wait . . . I take that back; G–d forbade its consumption at one integral point in the lives of man and woman. Actually, it was the first man and woman, to be exact. Adam and Eve ate from the forbidden fruit of the Tree of Life and committed the first sin. And then they covered themselves with fig leaves—"[t]hen the eyes of both were opened, and they knew that they were naked. And they sewed fig leaves together and made themselves loincloths" (Genesis 3:7). We are still reaping the consequences of the transgression!

Aside from the beginning of our creation, a plant-based diet with fresh fruits and vegetables is associated with a more positive real life in biblical times. Before Noah's time, the whole world ate a plant-based diet, which continued to be a large part of the agriculture lifestyle of the Israelites thereafter.

Fast-forward to our generation. Researchers have identified many plant benefits for our general health and weight loss. The media cannot wait to headline single attributes of the latest research—like the lycopene in a tomato—to ward off diseases and help us with memory. Reality is that a range of fruits and vegetables are shown to shield us against stroke and heart disease; control blood pressure; prevent different cancers; decrease the risk of developing cataracts and age-related macular degeneration, which can lead to vision loss; and also improve gut health, which prevents diverticulitis. In other words, they are delicious, G–d-given medications without side effects. You may then ask why I feel the need to address an important way to fulfill Steps Two and Three in my Steps to Living a Real Life with Real Food if we already know how beneficial fruit and veggies are for us. (Remember the steps state that you should eat *a lot* of vegetables and *some* fruit.).

Well, despite all the research behind fruits and vegetables, most of America is *still* not consuming enough! Statistics show less than 30 percent (1 in 3) of us are meeting the minimal recommendation to consume 5 to 13 servings of fruits and vegetables per day (2½ to 6½ cups per day), depending on your caloric needs.

More is better, especially when it comes to heart health. Those who do eat a minimum of 5 servings a day are 15 percent less likely to have a heart attack or other problems caused by restricted blood flow to the heart muscle than those who eat fewer servings per day. In the Nurse's Health Study (infamous research conducted by the Harvard School of Public Health that followed the health and dietary habits of 110,000 men and women for fourteen years), researchers found that the more produce a person consumed, the lower their risk of stroke—the third leading cause of death in the United States—and heart disease—the most serious form of cardiovascular disease that accounts for the most deaths in the United States per year. Conversely, those who ate a low amount of produce (1.5 cups per day) were found to have a higher risk than those who consumed 8 cups per day or more (which lessened their risk by 30 percent).[96] Further research confirmed those who ate more than 5 servings of fruits and vegetables experienced about a 2 percent lower risk of coronary heart disease[97] and stroke[98] compared to those who ate less than 3 servings per day. Wow! That is a lot of health protection.

Other studies also support the correlation between an increased fruit and vegetable intake with a reduction in coronary heart disease by 20 to 40 percent and stroke by 25 to 30 percent.[99] In particular, one study showed that cruciferous vegetables and citrus fruits had the most protective effects for heart disease, in addition to a high level of flavonoids, fiber, and folic acid, which may contribute to the protection against strokes.[100]

Each fruit and vegetable type has its own set of advantages and benefits to offer. For example, flavonoids, like quercetin, are phenols that are present in a variety of fresh produce and may help remove carcinogens from the body's cells. Isoflavones, a phytoestrogen, are uniquely found in one category of food known as legumes and appear to offer a protective effect by blocking binding to cell receptors; however, the effects of isoflavones on cancer are not so clear-cut (see chapter 8).

DISEASES AND CONDITIONS PREVENTED BY CONSUMPTION OF FRUITS AND VEGETABLES

CATARACTS

Cataracts are one of the leading causes of blindness. The caratenoids vitamin C and vitamin E in fruits and vegetables help to delay cataract formation.

CHRONIC OBSTRUCTIVE PULMONARY DISEASE (COPD)

A high intake of fruits and vegetables enhances ventilatory function, which reduces the risk of Chronic Obstructive Pulmonary Disease (COPD). Flavonoids, like quercetin, are generally contained in higher amounts in fruits than vegetables, particularly in their outer layers. Vitamin C is also cited as contributing to the protective effect against COPD. Not only is it an antioxidant, but it is also the main antioxidant found in the airway surface liquid of the lung, so it is located in a useful place to protect the body from harmful oxidants.

DIVERTICULOSIS

Diverticulosis is one of the most common conditions found in industrialized nations. The condition occurs when small pouches called diverticulum develop in the large intestine or colon. The diverticulum may remain asymptomatic but can lead to diverticulitis when the surrounding tissues become inflamed. This often occurs as a result of obstruction by dietary components or stool.

A high-fiber diet, which increases the bulk and moisture of the stool, reduces travel time through the gastrointestinal tract and contributes the highest protective effects against the development of diverticulosis. Researchers have found that the insoluble fiber, specifically the cellulose component from fruits and vegetables—not grains—reduces the risk of diverticulosis. Cellulose accounts for 30 percent of the insoluble fiber in fruits and 50 percent or more in vegetables. The other closest food with the highest amount of cellulose is legumes, and it accounts for half of total fiber.

HYPERTENSION

Hypertension afflicts about forty-three million Americans. Fruits and vegetables, about 8 to 10 servings per day, can lower blood pressure in people with or without hypertension. The high amount of potassium and magnesium in produce may also help to control hypertension.

CANCER

Cancer is the second leading cause of death after cardiovascular disease in the United States. Some of the strongest evidence supports the protective effects certain fruits and vegetables have on different types of cancer. More than 400 grams (more than 15 ounces) of fruit per day was found to prevent at least 20 percent of all incidences of cancer![101] Although the exact mechanisms are not understood, many of the protective benefits can be found in the different vitamins, minerals, dietary fiber, and other chemical components of the fruits and vegetables.

Benefits lie in the different *types* of produce. For example, the deep yellow and orange forms of produce are high in beta-carotene, a carotenoid; citrus fruits are high in vitamin C; leafy greens (especially spinach and collard) are high in lutein; and tomatoes are high in lycopene. All these components are antioxidants that protect cell membranes and DNA from oxidative damage.

Leafy greens are high in folic acid, which helps prevent cancer from a molecular level. Sulfur-containing compounds, like isothiocyanates and dithiolthiones, found abundantly in cruciferous vegetables like broccoli, cauliflower, and cabbage help increase enzyme activity involved in detoxifying carcinogens and other harmful substances. Also found in cruciferous vegetables are indoles, which are shown to block tumor production in animal studies. Onions, garlic, scallions, and leeks are in the allium family and contain sulfur compounds shown to activate enzyme detoxification systems in the body. So, basically, a wide array of fruits and vegetables attack cancer on many different levels, like an enemy walking into a mine field with booby traps; stepping on one sets off a cascade of explosions, but these explosions only serve to benefit our health.

HEART DISEASE

Similar beneficial effects on cancer are shown with heart disease. The antioxidants in fruits and vegetables from the sulfur-containing compounds of the allium family, along with antioxidant minerals zinc and selenium, prevent the oxidation of cholesterol in the arteries. Additionally, the folic acid present in green leafy vegetables, melons, and oranges along with vitamins B6 and B12 help to lower homocysteine, a known risk factor for cardiovascular disease. Finally, the soluble fiber helps to lower blood cholesterol levels, a risk factor for cardiovascular disease.

WEIGHT MANAGEMENT

Aside from the powerful protection against many diseases, fruits and vegetables aid in weight loss and weight management. First, they are very low in calories. Second, because of their high water and potassium content, they also help to flush your system and thus decrease swelling. Third, the high fiber components keep you fuller longer, which in turn causes you to eat less during the day, and because of the digestive rewards of fiber, helps you get a flatter tummy.

To live a real life with real food, incorporate vegetables as the main dish at both lunch and dinner and utilize fruits as part of your real-food snacks, fulfilling Steps Two and Three in the Steps to Living a Real Life with Real Food. As stated in chapter 3, when planning your meals, you should say, "I'll have XX vegetables with sides of XX starch and XX protein." Most of what you should be eating in your meal is vegetables.

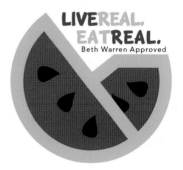

Tips for Eating More Fruits and Vegetables:

o **Breakfast:** Stir berries (fresh or frozen), dried fruit, or banana slices into yogurt, cereal, or oatmeal. Make a smoothie with 1 cup of fruit and some greens like cucumber, kale, or spinach. Make an egg omelet and grab some fresh or frozen veggies, like peppers, broccoli, and mushrooms to throw in.

o **Double the veggies in recipes.** Who says you only need ½ cup of broccoli? Stuff vegetables into sandwiches, make a pizza indulgence a better choice by piling vegetables on top, blend into casseroles (like a healthier mac and cheese recipe), or blend them into sauces . . . just get in the habit of always adding more!

o **Prep!** Make a large batch of fruit salad for the week (have about 1 cup at a time with a protein) or grill veggies and refrigerate.

o **Don't be fancy.** Roast string beans, asparagus, and other veggies for easy, fast, and delicious vegetable additions to your meal. No time to heat? Eat it raw! Crunch on some cucumbers for added veggies.

o **Get inspired.** Visit local farmers' markets and other specialty spots, or join a CSA (see CSA) to try one new vegetable a week.

o **Find the savings.** See which fruits and vegetables are in season and find the stores with sales so you can enjoy a budget-friendly meal.

o **Have it all around you.** Keep fresh fruits out on your desk or table at home. Precut and portion fresh fruits and vegetables and keep them on you.

o **Make a fresh green juice** to add to your meals or snacks.

o **Incorporate fruits into your dessert indulgences.** (See Recipes for dark chocolate with fruit and all-fruit ices.)

o **Experiment with salads.** Throw different fruits and veggies together and have them prepped in the fridge for easy and quick access.

o **Dip-In.** Make a platter of fresh vegetables and keep them nearby. Pair them with a healthy dip like hummus.

o **Use lettuce in place of bread as a wrap** around a protein like tuna.

Servings:

Rule of thumb for non-starchy produce is whatever you can fit in 1 cup as a serving. The exception is for leafy greens, which need to be filled into 2 cups to be the equivalent of a 1 cup serving. For dried fruit, I recommend a ¼ cup serving (½ cup filled with dried fruit equals 1 cup).

CSA

Community Supported Agriculture (CSA) became a popular way for consumers to buy local, seasonal food directly from a farmer. The way it works is a farmer offers a certain number of "shares" to the public—the "share" actually consists of a box of vegetables. Consumers purchase a membership that entitles them to receive a "share"—or box of seasonal produce the farmer picks out—during each week of the farming season. The benefits are similar to eating locally grown produce (see Local), but also adds a tantalizing challenge of cooking with new foods and tasting fruits and vegetables you may otherwise not have purchased.

GO ORGANIC?

The term *organic* has become ubiquitous—sort of like the term *kosher*. Many highly processed foods are masked under the term *organic* and people sometimes flock to purchase unhealthy cookies, cakes, and other products, all the while thinking they're automatically healthy. We constantly hear the debate on whether or not buying organic is truly better for one's health.

Typically, studies focus on the nutritional content. A recent Stanford Study published in the *Annals of Internal Medicine* in September 2012 garnered a lot of publicity with newsreels boasting headlines such as "Organic Food May Not Be Healthier for You." In a review of two hundred studies, the meta-analysis found that there was also no guarantee organic food would be pesticide-free, although it did have 30 percent lower levels compared to conventional products. Two studies of children consuming organic and conventional diets did find lower levels of pesticide residues in the urine of children on organic diets. Finally, the researchers did write that the "[c]onsumption of organic foods may reduce exposure to pesticide residues and antibiotic-resistant bacteria." So, it does seem that organic is actually better for you.

Some of the findings in the study missed the point of why people choose to go organic, though. There are other benefits to organic agriculture. According to Stonyfield.com, "Organic farmers and growers also don't handle toxic, persistent pesticides, herbicides, or chemical fertilizers that can pose a health hazard. Organic practices means livestock are kept strong, healthy, and productive through good nutrition, less stress, and humane living conditions, rather than through antibiotics or injections of artificial growth hormones. Our soil, rivers, drinking water, and air also benefit from organic agriculture because organic practices do not contaminate them with toxic-persistent chemicals. Organic means less dependence on fossil fuels and is estimated to have the same carbon-reducing effect as taking 217 million cars off the road!"

When it comes to fruits and vegetables, the issue of whether to eat non-organic supersedes the question of whether to eat fruits and vegetables if no organic options are available. Dr. David Servan-Schreiber wrote in his book *ANTICANCER*, "The fact that anticancer foods are able to detoxify bodies by eliminating carcinogens is particularly important. It follows, for example, that even if certain nonorganic fruits and vegetables are contaminated by pesticides, the powerful impact of anticancer molecules wins out over the negative effects of carcinogens." Plants were designed with survival mechanisms or phytonutrients, to ward off attack. We consume those protective components and rely on them to act the same way inside our bodies.

Organic produce has its benefits and you can try to eat organic in the most cost-effective way by following the Environmental Working Group's (EWG.com) annual list of the "Clean 15"—the produce with the least pesticides—and the "Dirty Dozen"—the produce sprayed with the highest amount of pesticides:

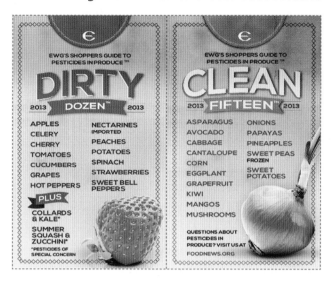

So What's the Deal with Organic?

Organic foods account for 4.2 percent of retail food sales, according to the US Department of Agriculture (USDA). The USDA certifies products as organic if they are produced without synthetic pesticides or fertilizers or routine use of antibiotics or growth hormones. We pay a lot more for some organic products, mostly because these farms are not subsidized by the government, but demand is increasing. Organic foods accounted for $31.4 billion sales in 2011, according to an Obama administration report, up from $3.6 billion in 1997.

Phytonutrients: What are they?

I love when patients come in and spew fancy terms and words like "phytonutrients." When I ask them what the word means, they are dumbfounded. Allow me to explain: Phytochemicals have antioxidant abilities, which means they can help neutralize free radicals in the body that might otherwise damage cells. As a result, they help prevent or reduce symptoms of some types of diseases. They act as messengers in the body, functioning similarly to hormones.

The chemical composition of a fruit or vegetable, including its phytonutrients, vary with the season, the soil it grew in, how much water it received, which bugs it had to withstand, how ripe it was when it was picked and eaten, and the storage conditions. Hundreds of components are still being discovered, along with the interplay between the different complex compounds and their effects on our health, which is one reason why vitamin supplements are not as effective as eating the whole fruit and why eating a variety is a key factor in achieving good overall health.

LOCAL

A movement has been made by a group known as *locavores*—people committed to eating locally grown foods, a practice which contributes a lot to your health, the environment, and your tastebuds! Because of the freshness from the short transition from the farm to your table, food is tastier and has a smaller chance of losing key nutrients during long transit. Also, you can develop a rapport with a farmer in close-to-home places such as farmers' markets, enabling you to trust the source and safety of your food. If you are looking to lower the toxic load in your body, most local farmers explain they use minimal pesticides, so their produce is not as exposed as conventionally grown produce shipped from further distances. And it's a great deed to shop locally, since you are helping to support local farmers and sustain agricultural lands and lifestyles, build community, conserve fertile soil and clean water, and build a better habitat for animals.

So What's the Deal with GMOs?

Genetically Engineering (GE) or Genetic Modification (GM) of food is a process of artificially inserting genes into the DNA of food crops or animals. The genes can come from bacteria, viruses, insects, animals, or even humans. The result is a genetically modified organism, or GMO. The United States, unlike many other industrialized countries, does not require labeling of GMOs.

Research is in the relatively early stages on the effects of GMO on the quality of food, the environment, and our health. It is disconcerting that food manufacturers are not forthcoming with using GMO ingredients, as consumers have the right to know what is in their food. Until GMO ingredients are publicized, you can limit your exposure to GMO products by trying the following whenever possible:

- Go Organic. The organic labeled products require only 70 percent of the ingredients be organic, but 100 percent must be non-GMO.
- Look for voluntary labels that read non-GMO or MADE WITHOUT GENETICALLY MODIFIED INGREDIENTS. Some companies place these on their products or next to questionable ingredients like soy lecithin.
- Avoid the big four: processed foods made with corn, soybeans, canola, and cottonseed, which may look like these within the ingredient list:

  Corn

    o Corn flour, meal, oil, starch, gluten, and syrup
    o Sweeteners such as fructose, dextrose, and glucose
    o Modified food starch*

Soy

  o   Soy flour, lecithin, protein, isolate, and isoflavone

  o   Vegetable oil* and vegetable protein*

Canola oil (also called rapeseed oil)

Cottonseed oil

*May be derived from other sources

- Look for Non-GMO cane sugar or organic and non-GMO sweeteners, candy, and chocolate products made with 100 percent cane sugar, evaporated cane juice, or organic sugar to avoid GM beet sugar.[102]

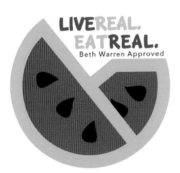

Our goal of living a real life with real food is to limit heavily processed foods for many other reasons, so you will naturally limit GMO exposure as well when adopting a fresher, more real food lifestyle.

SOMETHING TO THINK ABOUT: FERMENTATION

Fermenting vegetables, or pickling, has become a popular trend today. The process, referred to as *lacto-fermentation*, metabolizes natural sugars in fruits and vegetables and, under the right circumstances, creates lactic acid, enzymes, antioxidants, and vitamins. Lacto-fermentation has been shown to improve the nutritional value and digestibility of these foods.[103]

Aside from providing a signature sour taste, the process allows for live beneficial bacteria, or cultures, to grow. When you consume them, they help to ward off harmful bacteria in the gut, digest food, absorb nutrients, and regulate our immune system (see Benefits of Lactic Acid Bacteria).

But the art of fermentation, or pickling (which is called turshi), is nothing new. It was an intrinsic part of not only my Middle Eastern history, but others as well. During medieval times, most cultures consumed fermented foods and vegetables: it was called kimchi in Korea, zuke in Japan, chutneys in India, and pickled cabbage in China. The Sephardic Jewry in Spain adopted the art of pickling vegetables from the Iberian culture. Pickles and relishes became an essential part of the diet, from the impoverished to the wealthy—not only for the health benefits, but also the enhancement in color, flavor, and texture to meals. These attributes contributed an undeniable palatability to the usual bland meal of hard-bread.[104]

Incorporating pickled dishes was also a part of keeping Jewish laws. The Talmud (collection of Jewish laws and traditions consisting of the Mishnah and Gemara) states, "One who is about to recite the Hamotzi (blessing over bread) is not allowed to do so until salt and leaften (relish) is placed before him." The Hebrew word *leaften* came from the word *Lefet*, meaning turnip, which was derived from the word *lefhet*, which meant to twist and turn when referring to the way a root vegetable is harvested. Turnips are one of the most popular vegetables typically fermented and are still displayed on the Sabbath at my table. *Leaften* refers to most relishes, though, and was always an accompaniment to bread at Middle Eastern meals.

At first, the pickling in Spain relied on vinegar, primarily from wine, to ferment vegetables. But in Eastern Europe, wine was hard to come by. They adapted the more advanced form of fermentation from China, the lacto-fermentation associated with numerous health benefits.

Lacto-fermentation does not use any vinegar, but instead relies on the acidifying bacteria inherently found in a raw vegetable that feeds off its natural sugars. Just the right amount of salt is also an important ingredient for protecting against harmful bacteria and extrapolating the water and sugar from the vegetables. If there is too much salt, it will not ferment. Lacto-fermentation also needs warm, moist conditions to be successful. During fermentation, the vegetables produce lactic and acetic acids, which soften the vegetables and give a tangy, "pickled" flavor.

As the art of lacto-fermentation spread throughout European Jews, the staple sauerkraut, or raw cabbage, was born. The store-bought packaged sauerkraut of today does not reap the benefits of the lacto-fermented products of the old days because the modern-day process of pasteurization kills the beneficial bacteria, as well. (See Recipes for making your own raw cabbage and other fermented vegetables.) Other vegetables typically fermented are beets, carrots, cauliflower, mushrooms, olives, cucumbers, peppers, green tomatoes, and turnips.

Barrels of fermented cucumbers can still be seen in many pickle stores, especially in Lower Manhattan. They are referred to as *kosher dills* and have a signature sour flavor. Today, they're made with fresh garlic. My grandmother, Sarah, was an Ashkenazi Jew of Eastern European decent, who was married to a Sephardic Jew, my grandfather, Al, who was the son of parents from Aleppo and Damascus, Syria. Her cooking reflected the clash of two cultures. Lining her countertops were jars of all sizes with vegetables like peppers, turnips, and green tomatoes packed inside, fermenting and waiting for tasting. When she visited, I could depend on her to bring two things: fresh apple sauce and pickled vegetables, usually peppers, in large mason jars. She passed away in 2009, but her jars and the old-fashioned food mill she used to grind applesauce were two pieces of her life I kept with me . . . and with my kitchen.

Benefits of Lactic Acid Bacteria

o   Reduces the levels of anti-nutrients such as phytic acid and tannins in food, leading to increased bioavailability of minerals such as iron, protein, and simple sugars

o   Increases the amount of vitamins in the fermented food

o   Acts as a form of detoxification that preserves the nutritive value and flavor of decontaminated food. In addition to this, lactic acid bacteria fermentation irreversibly degrades mycotoxins without leaving any toxic residues.

o   Shown to have anti-tumor effects

o   Prevents diarrheal diseases because they modify the composition of intestinal microorganisms, and by this, act as deterrents for pathogenic enteric bacteria

o   Produces fungal inhibitory metabolites. These are mainly organic acids, which include propionic, acetic and lactic acids.

o   Produces protein antimicrobial agents such as bacteriocins. Bacteriocins are peptides that elicit antimicrobial activity against food spoilage organisms and food borne pathogens, but do not affect the producing organisms.

o   Synthesizes other antimicrobial compounds, such as hydrogen peroxide, reuterin, and reutericyclin

o   Works as probiotics that restore the gut flora in patients suffering from diarrhea, following usage of antibiotics that destroy the normal flora. In this manner, fermented food is used to prevent and to alleviate diarrhea.

o   Alleviates constipation and abdominal cramps.

We may have gotten a bit heavy in research surrounding fruits and vegetables, but this is because the results are crystal clear and show they can benefit anyone and everyone. The more you eat, the merrier (and healthier) you'll be! Although each fruit and vegetable has its own great attributes, and it is

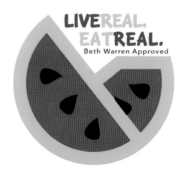

important to eat a variety of colors to consume each benefit, incorporating a higher amount of dark green leafy, cruciferous and yellow-orange vegetables, along with citrus and deep yellow orange fruits, show the highest links to protecting you and preventing the diseases associated with oxidative damage including cancers, cardiovascular disease, stroke, cataracts, and COPD. The most notable protective elements are vitamin C, flavonoids, and carotenoids along with the sulfur-containing compounds in the allium family of vegetables (which are especially helpful in preventing heart disease) and the dithiothiones, indoles, and disothiocyanates in cruciferous vegetables (which aid in the prevention of cancer).

Ultimately, if you are going to try to live a life with real food, benefit your health, and reach your weight-loss goals, you will need to incorporate a large proportion of fruits and vegetables into your daily intake. **Remember:** A lot of vegetables. Some fruit.

The statistics make it clear that even if you support this idea, you most likely still needed some convincing before reading this chapter. Hopefully, with my highlights on the benefits of the fruits and vegetables most frequently consumed in my Middle Eastern and Eastern European roots, in addition to my ideas for ways to enjoy them (not to mention reminders about what research shows regarding their benefits to your health and goals of weight loss), you will be encouraged to incorporate them more into your real life. Be sure to also check out some real food recipes (see Recipes) for ideas on how to translate each fruit or vegetable into an actual, real life, dish.

CHAPTER 8

PROTEIN—QUALITY VERSUS QUANTITY

*"And G–d said, 'Behold, I have given you every plant yielding
seed that is on the face of all the earth, and every tree with seed
in its fruit. You shall have them for food.'"*

—*Genesis 1:29*

Protein is a vital nutrient that plays a significant role in your health. It is responsible for keeping your skin and hair healthy and muscles strong. Protein is the last nutrient on your path toward eating real food for your real life because most people already get an adequate supply, overall, since protein is in most foods. Another reason is because some of the proteins I will highlight are not necessarily from my Jewish roots. Although common in our modern-day cuisine, they are not all unique to our culture. Of course, this nutritious and delicious nutrient is no stranger to controversy.

As you have read through the chapters, the theme of a real life with real food diet stresses *quality* food. Deciphering between high-quality proteins has its own set of confusion because we do not necessarily absorb all the protein in a food.

AMINO ACID TYPES

Essential	Nonessential
Histidine	Alanine
Isoleucine	Arginine*
Leucine	Aspartic acid
Lysine	Cysteine*
Methionine	Glutamic acid
Phenylalanine	Glutamine*
Threonine	Glycine*
Tryptophan	Proline*
Valine	Serine*
	Tyrosine*
	Asparagine*
	Selenocysteine

Most non-essential amino acids (the building blocks of protein) are from a storage pool inside our bodies, but we burn through them more quickly than our fat stores. Other essential amino acids need to be consumed from food. The "starred" amino acids in the chart (see Essential versus Nonessential) are considered "conditionally essential," which means under specific situations or in certain areas of deficiencies, they become essential:

Dangers of Too Much Protein (Supplements)

Louis was a poster child for physical activity. He hit the gym nightly, never missing one day of exercise. Over time, Louis's love for the gym turned into an unhealthy obsession with bodybuilding. As a result, he put himself on multiple supplements for what he thought (and was promised by marketing messages and fellow gym-goers) would aid in his muscle-building goals.

When he started his gym obsession, Louis was clinically obese. Not from the weight of muscle, but he had body fat that he needed to lose. The addition of amino acid supplements, which are not needed, would turn into fat. Even worse, the overuse of supplements can become detrimental to your health.

It is excellent to engage in physical activity, but only when it is in a healthy way with realistic goals that fall in line with what your individual body needs. Louis is one of many patients who asked about protein supplements to help them build muscle faster. But most supplements are unnecessary, unproven, and unregulated by the FDA. Not to mention, some are dangerous, so proceed with caution and ask for advice from an expert registered dietitian, not your local friends at the gym.

Protein is absolutely necessary to building muscle, but too much protein can harm your body. One way proteins can be harmful is through digestion. Calcium and other components help neutralize the acids formed by digesting the protein in a food, but if you consume too much protein, your body will begin to pull calcium mainly from your bones, the largest storage inside your body. In the Nurses' Health Study, women who ate 95 grams of protein (more than 25 percent of their daily calories), reported more broken wrists than those consuming a more moderate amount of 68 grams of protein (less than 15 percent of daily calories).

While there are dangers of eating too much protein, the importance of a protein-rich diet in context of other whole foods is huge. It helps with your weight-loss goals in a few key ways:

1. Protein increases your fullness to a greater extent than fat and carbohydrates, and therefore, may cause you to eat fewer calories per meal.
2. Eating relatively more protein increases thermogenesis, your body's way of burning calories while processing it, which may help promote a feeling of fullness.
3. A protein-rich diet helps maintain muscle while you are trying to lose weight. Diets that promote rapid weight loss or restrict protein (such as the fad "juice fasts") cause a loss in muscle, not fat, which does not benefit you in the long run and slows down your metabolic rate.[105]

SOURCES OF PROTEIN

Here are some great sources of protein that should grab your attention:

LOVING LEGUMES

Legumes, frequently consumed as part of Middle Eastern and Mediterranean meals, are great additions to your diet for their rich source of folate, fiber, magnesium, and iron as well as their protecting phytonutrients anthocyanins and quercetin. Packed with these antioxidants and more, their color is a G–d given map toward benefitting different aspects of our health. They are shown to protect against coronary heart disease, diabetes, high blood pressure, and inflammation.

The legume family includes alfalfa, clover, lupins, green beans and peas, peanuts, soybeans, dry beans, broad beans, dry peas, chickpeas, and lentils. Here are a few legumes that are my go-to plant-based proteins:

BEANS

Beans, referenced in both the books of Ezekiel and Samuel, can fit into any of the featured food groups on your plate. They have starch and protein and are a vegetable, too. High in both soluble and insoluble fiber, beans help to promote a healthy digestive tract, which minimizes the risk of gut-related conditions and some types of cancer. They also help lower cholesterol and improve insulin sensitivity, decreasing the risk for heart disease and diabetes.

Beans contain a variety of vitamins and minerals including calcium, phosphorus, potassium, folate, magnesium, and iron. Calcium and phosphorus play a vital role in bone health; potassium works with sodium to maintain healthy blood pressure; folate is a B vitamin that is often associated with healthy pregnancy. It is also necessary for the production and maintenance of new cells. Magnesium has many purposes: it is needed for muscle and nerve function, a healthy immune system, bone health, blood pressure regulation, and energy metabolism. Finally, iron is an important part of oxygen-transporting proteins within the blood and it also promotes cell growth.

Beans have a high phytic acid content, so it is best to soak your beans for twenty-four hours to minimize the effects of interfering with some vitamin and mineral absorption (see chapter 6). If you are short on time and need to use canned beans, be sure to give them a good rinse prior to use because of their high sodium content. Also, try to use brands with

BPA-free (bisephenol A) lining, like Eden® Foods. I also recommend not adding any sodium to the dish because some salt remains on the beans post-washing.

Sometimes, the high fiber content may leave you feeling bloated and gassy. Try to consume beans slowly at first, with one half-cup serving, keep your intake consistent, and drink water with each dish. Do not be afraid to experiment with all kinds of beans in your cooking, as they add a palatable, visually stimulating, and satisfying aspect to your dish. If you are vegan or vegetarian, it is even more crucial you consume many forms of beans.

LOTS OF LENTILS

Through my Syrian heritage, I learned to incorporate lentils in soups, with rice, and as a cold salad. But the connection between lentils and Judaism has a deeply rooted importance in our diets.

Jacob gave Esau, his brother, lentil stew he cooked after his grandfather, Abraham, passed away (a custom to cook Ades soup is based on this historical event. See Recipes.) in exchange for Esau's birthright. He then tricked his father, Isaac, with a stew and won his brother's blessing (Genesis 25:29).

The nutritional quality of all lentils are superb: one cup of cooked lentils contains about 18 grams of protein, 15 grams of fiber, over 6 mg of iron, 38 mg of calcium, and is a good source of potassium and magnesium. Lentils also have vitamin C and K, which are important for blood clotting. They also contain small amounts of zinc, selenium, and copper.[106]

GARBANZO BEANS (AKA CHICKPEAS)

Chickpeas are another prominent food in my Middle Eastern culture. It's a good thing, too, because a 100-gram serving of cooked garbanzo beans without salt contains 27.42 grams carbohydrates; 7.6 grams dietary fiber; 2.59 grams fat; and 8.86 grams of protein. One half-cup serving of cooked garbanzo beans has 2.37 mg of iron, meeting 13 percent of your daily value, and 141 mcg of folate, meeting 35 percent of your recommended daily value.

Garbanzo beans also contain vitamin A, thiamine, riboflavin, niacin, pantothenic acid, vitamin B6, folate, and vitamins C, E, and K. Chickpeas also have the minerals calcium, iron, magnesium, phosphorus, potassium, sodium, and zinc.

A study conducted in 2010 showed that chickpeas can also control your hunger. A group of forty-two participants maintained their normal diet for four weeks, then added 104 grams of garbanzo beans for twelve weeks, and completed the study with their normal diet, without the beans, for an additional four weeks. While the participants were eating the garbanzo beans, they ate fewer calories overall and reported an increase in satiation—a great way to help manage your weight!

A similar study in 2007 compared a diet with garbanzo beans versus one supplemented with high-fiber wheat foods and their effects on blood cholesterol levels. After only five weeks, participants saw a reduction with both diets, but a significantly greater percentage in total cholesterol and LDL cholesterol during the chickpea diet than during the high-fiber wheat diet.[107]

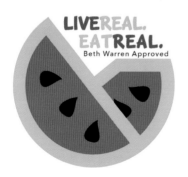

I stamp my Kosher Seal of Approval on all variants of the legume family. From black, to kidney, to navy beans, each has their own set of nutritional value for our health. For fresh beans, soak them overnight. For canned, give them a rinse before using. Keep in mind that beans account for both starch and protein. When you make your plate, be sure to reserve beans to one-quarter of your plate, about a half-cup, as a starch. If beans are the protein and you are eating another starch, you can eat one-cup of beans. If you are not eating another protein or a starch at a meal, you can expand your beans to cover half your plate, so they can attribute more protein and starch to your meal.

Did You Know?

Did you know that string beans are the only "bean" that does not count as a starch? String beans can be equivalent to half your plate at each meal. They are a good source of B vitamins and vitamin C, which help to build your immune system, as well as fiber (1.6 g in a half-cup), folate, vitamin K, vitamin A, protein, and calcium (31.5 mg per a half-cup). Yum![108]

THE SUPER EGG

The egg industry's marketing tagline, "The Incredible, Edible Egg," could not be more on point. Jam-packed with essential vitamins and minerals, and only about 76 calories per large egg, this quality animal protein (6.3 grams each) is a great addition to your diet. Too bad the low-fat craze hurt its reputation. Scientists clustered eggs as contributors of an increase in cholesterol and heart disease. As a result, many eliminated the vital food source from our diets. Since we already accomplished the necessity of healthy fats in our diets, let us see how else an egg can help us achieve a real life with real food.

YOLK VERSUS WHITE

Egg whites do offer more protein than the yolk (as well as most of the magnesium, potassium, niacin, and sodium), but they do not contain anywhere near the quantity of vitamins in the yolk. Egg whites have fewer calories, totaling about 17 per egg compared to 59 in the yolk.

The frequently disposed of egg yolk is actually the only place you will find the beneficial fat-soluble vitamins A, E, D, and K and more than 90 percent of the vitamins B6 and B12. The egg white became synonymous with the protein of the egg, but the yolk contains nearly half the protein of the whole egg. Yolks also contain more than 90 percent of the calcium, iron, phosphorus, zinc, thiamin, folate, and fat of the egg.

Maybe now you will think twice before you throw that yolk in the garbage?

SPOTLIGHT ON CHOLINE

Egg yolks are a great source of choline, a B vitamin. Unfortunately, 90 percent of Americans are deficient in this vital nutrient, primarily because it is not found in most foods and our bodies do not make enough of it. A choline deficiency leads to a deficiency in another key B vitamin, folic acid.

Choline is a vital component in brain health. It is integral to all the body's fat-containing structures and cell membranes, including both phosphatidylcholine and sphingomyelin, two fat-like molecules that account for a large percentage of the total mass in the brain.

Choline has three methyl groups and is, therefore, important in methylation, a process in which methyl groups are transferred from one to another, similar to cells sending messages back and forth. Both choline and betaine, its by-product found in foods like beets and soybeans, work together in the cellular process of methylation, which is not only responsible for the removal of homocysteine, but is involved in turning off the promoter regions of genes involved in inflammation. Acting as a huge anti-inflammatory agent, consumption of choline is linked with a decrease in heart disease, osteoporosis, cognitive decline and Alzheimer's, and type-2 diabetes.

Choline helps comprise acetylcholine, a neurotransmitter that brings messages to and from nerves and muscles—the primary way your body sends messages. It is also linked to lower anxiety because of choline's important role within the central nervous system.

Your Heart on Eggs

Aside from choline's affect on your brain and nervous system, it also improves cardiovascular health by helping convert homocysteine, a molecule that has potential to damage blood vessels, into more benign substances. Additionally, the egg's quality source of vitamin B12 enhances the process of converting homocysteine into safer molecules.

The cholesterol in the egg, or more specifically, the yolk, is one of the major factors that gives eggs a bad name. But now, even the American Heart Association says that, based on multiple studies, those on a low-fat diet can eat one or two eggs a day without measurable changes in their blood cholesterol levels. One study found that saturated fat in the diet, not dietary cholesterol, is what influences blood cholesterol levels the most. Another study showed eggs actually improve the lipid (cholesterol) profile by changing the type of cholesterol in the body. After a month of eating two eggs daily, not only did it not negatively affect the ratio of LDL:HDL, but it also increased the size of the LDL cholesterol—a significant change since larger LDL is much less atherogenic (likely to promote atherosclerosis) versus the smaller LDL particles.[109]

Eggs and Weight Loss

Most of your goals to lose fat include losing belly fat, and choline is shown to be a belly-blaster. Researchers showed that the group who ate eggs versus people who ate a bagel for breakfast for five days lost twice as much weight in eight weeks; an average of six pounds more than the bagel eaters.[110] They also had an 85 percent greater decrease in waist circumference and reported greater improvements in energy. Both groups positively showed no difference in triglyceride or total cholesterol or HDL and LDL levels.[111]

LUTEIN: AN ANTIOXIDANT

Lutein—a carotenoid thought to help prevent age-related macular degeneration and cataracts—may be found in even higher amounts in eggs than in green vegetables. Produce such as spinach were once considered lutein's major dietary sources. When found in eggs, lutein is better absorbed than in green vegetables and even supplements. One study showed that after five weeks of eating a daily egg, participants' blood levels of lutein and zeaxanthin significantly increased by 26 percent and 38 percent, respectively, compared to their levels of these carotenoids after their no-egg week.

Lutein, like other carotenoids, is fat soluble, so it cannot be absorbed unless fat is also present. Being fat soluble is also the case with vitamins A, E, D, and K—all found in the egg yolk, and therefore, better absorbed due to their good company of healthy fats.

I hope I intrigued your taste buds and that you're now convinced that you should try to incorporate more eggs into your diet. Here's some ideas of how to do just that:

- Try a poached or scrambled egg for breakfast
- Prepare an egg salad sandwich for work
- Include a hard-boiled egg for a snack

WHICH EGGS ARE BEST?

Eggs are no different than most other food groups that got caught up in marketing frenzy. From organic, to cage-free, free-range, and vegetable-fed (literally meaning they were fed a vegetarian-based diet), the many terms describing the quality of eggs leave consumers scratching their heads in confusion of which to buy.

Organic Eggs

Simply stating something is organic does not tell us what food the chickens were fed (which determines the nutritional composition of the egg);

it only tells us that it was organic. As with most animal proteins, organic means their feed was organic and they were not given antibiotics or hormones. Organic chickens may be left uncaged but are not required to have outdoor access and typically stay inside the barn or warehouse.

Cage-Free

Unfortunately, when an egg carton lists the term *cage-free*, it only requires a chicken to be out of their cage for at least five minutes, and there is no specificity on *where* they should be when outside their cage. It may mean the chickens are still roaming in their dark, crowded, indoor coup.

Free-Range

Free-range means that the chickens can roam on green pastures, unlimited, yet the label requires they have a minimum of five minutes outside per day, without specifics on duration or quality. It also does not guarantee the chicken actually got outside because most hen houses have a small hole in the coop that one of many chickens has to cram through. This means that some simply stay indoors. When, and if, the chicken finally has access to the "outdoors," it can be a grass field or a section of hard-core pavement.

Pastured Eggs

The accurate term to describe the quality eggs we all should seek out is *pastured*. There is no federal definition of pastured eggs, and it is difficult to find them. More than likely, you will encounter them at some specialty health-food stores and local farmers' market, which is a great place to find a farmer you can trust to get quality pastured eggs.

Being pastured-raised, the chickens are cage-free all day and roam the fields to eat green plants and insects. At night, they go back to their hen house, roost, and lay eggs. During the winter months, they may be supplemented with organic feed. The quality of pastured eggs may also be more nutritious: more vitamin D, vitamin A, vitamin E, Omega-3 fatty acids, and beta-carotene.

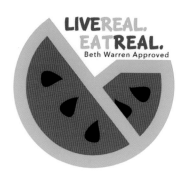

If pastured eggs are not available, look for the words, "organic, cage-free, Omega-3" on the carton, which includes eggs layed from a hen fed a diet rich in flaxseed. These eggs are a good source of not only of lutein and zeaxanthin, but also Omega-3 essential fatty acids. One study found that Omega-3 eggs contain 39 percent less Arachidonic Acid (AA), an Omega-6 fat that promotes inflammation, than only conventional or organic. Furthermore, they are rich in different types of Omega-3 fats, both the short- and long-chains. Omega-3 eggs are certainly not nutritionally equivalent to pastured eggs, but they're a step in the right direction.[112] They also guarantee that, at the very least, the chickens/hens were not given any antibiotics or hormones. Keep in mind that the color of the outer shell tells us nothing about the nutritional quality or value of the egg.

Grading By Quality and Size

The US Department of Agriculture grades eggs by the interior quality of the egg and the appearance and condition of the eggshell. Eggs of any quality grade may differ in weight (size).

o   US Grade AA

- Eggs have whites that are thick and firm; yolks that are high, round, and practically free from defects; and clean, unbroken shells. Grade AA and Grade A eggs are best for frying and poaching, where appearance is important.

o US Grade A

- Eggs have characteristics of Grade AA eggs except the whites are "reasonably" firm. This is the quality most often sold in stores.

o US Grade B

- Eggs have whites that may be thinner and yolks that may be wider and flatter than eggs of higher grades. The shells must be unbroken, but may show slight stains.

    This quality is seldom found in retail stores because they are usually used to make liquid, frozen, and dried egg products, as well as other egg-containing products.

Source: http://en.wikipedia.org/wiki/Egg_(food)

FISH

Fish—especially the kosher varieties of salmon, sardines, herring, and tuna—have a great protein level, low saturated fat content, and quality vitamins, like vitamin D.

They are applauded for their high level of quality Omega-3 fats, the most readily absorbed form of EPA (eicosapentanoic acid) and DHA (docosahexapentanoic acid). Your body absorbs these forms of Omega-3s efficiently. This is unlike the way the body absorbs ALA (alpha-linolenic acid), found in other delicious and healthful plant-based sources such as leafy greens, walnuts, chia and flaxseeds, which need to be broken down to DHA/EPA by the liver before it can be absorbed and most is lost in the process.

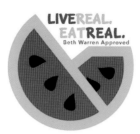

TYPE OF KOSHER FISH	TOTAL OMEGA-3 CONTENT PER 3.5 OUNCES (GRAMS)
Trout, lake	2.0
Herring	1.7
Tuna, bluefin	1.6
Salmon	1.5
Sardines, canned	1.5
Tuna, albacore	1.5
Whitefish, lake	1.5
Anchovies	1.4
Bluefish	1.2
Bass, striped	0.8
Trout, brook	0.6
Trout, rainbow	0.6
Halibut, Pacific	0.5
Pollock	0.5
Bass, fresh water	0.3
Flounder	0.2
Haddock	0.2
Snapper, red	0.2
Sole	0.1

SOURCE: THE HEALTH EFFECTS OF POLYUNSATURATED FATTY ACIDS IN SEAFOODS

WILD VERSUS FARMED

Wild seafood is a true organic protein source. These fish were born and bred in their natural aquatic environment. They have not been tampered with through feeding or medicinal or scientific methods. As a result, they may show higher levels of mercury than farmed fish. Typically, wild Alaskan salmon is a great and safe choice because it is low in mercury and high in Omega-3 fats, EPA and DHA, B6, B12, zinc, copper, selenium, vitamin D, helping to boost mood, fight cancer, and build strong bones. A great website to check aquatic situations in your area and for information on oil spills or other environmental impacts that may affect the quality of your wild fish is epa.gov.

When fish are farmed, they are born and/or raised in enclosures or tanks for commercial use. They may be given anything from growth hormones and antibiotics to corn and soy feed, both high in Omega-6 fats that can potentially change your fish from being anti- to pro-inflammatory! They may also have higher PCB and dioxin contamination levels.

Take caution when choosing fish and be mindful about the amount you eat per week because of high mercury levels (about 8 to 12 oz per week, according to the FDA and EPA). That being said, many varieties can be enjoyed, both in taste and health, in a kosher, real-food diet. When some patients express their dislike of the "fishy" taste, I often find they are not preparing fish well. See Recipes for ways to prepare fish and fit the time to prepare it into your real life.

Anchovies and Sardines

Although not usually a fan favorite, eating little wild fish such as anchovies and sardines is a great boost to your nutrition profile. These tiny creatures are high in Omega-3 fatty acids, protein,

B vitamins, iron, phosphorus, potassium, and the compound DMAE, which may improve brain function—and they're good for our oceans, as well. Because they are low on the food chain, you do not have to worry about consuming mercury either.

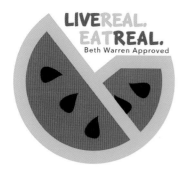

I have read conflicting opinions on which ways of breeding have higher compositions of Omega-3s, but because of all the other manhandling with farmed fish, I stick with the wild, or what I call *real* fish, whenever possible. In the kosher world, it is difficult to find many wild fish varieties, and they have a higher price tag. Either direction you decide to turn, eating low mercury fish with higher Omega-3 gets my Kosher Seal of Approval, whether you go for wild or farmed.

There are kosher dietary restrictions when it comes to fish. Only fish with fins and scales are kosher. Therefore, some fish high in Omega-3 (and happens to also be high in mercury) are unkosher including swordfish, mackerel, tilefish, and all shellfish.

SOY

Out of all the food discussed throughout the book, soy has been the most difficult to find the truth about while sifting through all the controversy. The reason is simple: both sides are so extreme. Either you support soy or are against it. I cannot simply say, "Eat it, because, if anything, it may benefit but will not harm," because those against soy consumption bring up scary effects of soy on our health. So, I researched and read through the different sides, wrote and rewrote this section as new evidence came to light, and even flip-flopped the sides I was taking.

All the while, feeling so sorry for you, the consumer, who may be more confused than I am!

THE BASICS

First, we will start with the basics of soy. Soybeans are a legume and a plant from the pea family. They are high in quality protein and are known to be an effective substitution for meat protein, which aids in weight loss. A research analysis showed that when participants switched their red meat and dairy consumption to soy, they had a higher intake of folate, vitamin K, calcium, magnesium, iron, and fiber. Soy is also high in the minerals copper, manganese, molybdenum, phosphorous, and potassium, the B vitamin riboflavin, and the Omega-3 form of ALA. Because of their plant-based properties and inherently lower level of saturated fat, they are shown to help decrease blood pressure and cholesterol. In fact, because of the research that suggests a daily intake of soy protein may slightly lower levels of LDL ("bad") cholesterol, the FDA came up with their own stamp of health approval for soy in 1999:

> "25 grams of soy protein a day, as part of a diet low in saturated fat and cholesterol, may reduce the risk of heart disease."

Other sides warn against the wide use of soy and argue the beneficial results are not as clear-cut.[113] In 2006, the American Heart Association (AHA), and many other researchers, disputed the FDA's claims in a study investigating the research on soy and wrote:

> "In the majority of 22 randomized trials, isolated soy protein with isoflavones, as compared with milk or other proteins, decreased LDL cholesterol concentrations… approximately 3%. This reduction is very small relative to the large amount of soy protein tested in these studies,

averaging 50 g, about half the usual total daily protein intake. No significant effects on HDL cholesterol, triglycerides, lipoprotein(a), or blood pressure were evident. Among 19 studies of soy isoflavones, the average effect on LDL cholesterol and other lipid risk factors was nil."

Throughout history, soy has also been used to treat menopausal symptoms, such as hot flashes. The same AHA study concluded soy was not shown to lessen these symptoms and had mixed results on its effects on soy's ability to slow postmenopausal bone loss. The finding is pretty much the consensus: there are no clear links between soy and its effects on menopausal symptoms.

For cancer, the AHA reported the efficacy and safety of soy isoflavones for preventing or treating cancer of the breast, endometrium, and prostate was not established and cautioned a possible adverse effect. They, therefore, did not recommend soy food or pills in treatment.

The reality is the research surrounding soy and cancer is perhaps the most controversial. Many studies show that genistein, the isoflavone phytonutrient in soy (see Isoflavones) is a key factor in cancer-prevention. Genistein is shown to increase the activity of the tumor suppressor protein called p53. When p53 becomes more active, it triggers apoptosis (programmed cell death) in cancer cells and inhibits activity of the cancer cells. It may also help slow tumor formation by blocking the protein kinases, especially in the case of breast cancers. However, in women with breast cancer who are premenopausal and have developed tumors that are neither estrogen-receptor or progesterone-receptor positive, intake of soy and genistein did not seem to lower the risk. In the end, it seems other dietary factors, for example, affect the benefits of soy. For example, if a person is not consuming enough fruits and vegetables, soy foods may not provide anticancer benefits.

In other cases, there is evidence that a large amount of processed soy parts—for example, dietary supplementation of soy isoflavones—may increase certain cancers such as breast cancer.

The overall negative effects are expected from antioxidants that act as an anti-tumor and anti-inflammatory agent, in any food, not just in soy. The same helpful components can become pro-oxidant, pro-inflammatory, and pro-tumor under certain conditions. The ying-yang affect of truly positive to dangerously negative is where the soy controversy gets its heat.

Finally, the AHA study concluded with:

> "The benefits of soy products on cardiovascular and over-all health should be attributed to their high content of polyunsaturated fats, fiber, vitamins, and minerals and low content of saturated fat as is the case with most other legumes and not specific to soy."[114]

Dr. Walter Willet of the Harvard School of Public Health also points out in his book, *Eat, Drink, and Be Healthy*, that the evidence on soy benefits and heart health is weak and the large amount of soy connected with the reported benefits is in conjunction with a high intake of saturated fat, which does not offset the risks of having too much saturated fat in the diet.

SOY AND INFLAMMATION

Originating from the Asian diets, which incorporated the whole soybean in small amounts, modern-day American food manufacturers have taken soy as one of their own, most often cracking, dehulling, crushing, or subjecting it to solvent extraction processes to separate the oils from the rest of the bean and molding them into ingredients for heavily processed foods.

Soybean oil has a more of the pro-inflammatory, Omega-6 level of polyunsaturated fat versus the Omega-3 levels (an Omega-3:Omega-6 ratio of 1:7). Because of its overuse in most processed foods, it is estimated that 10 percent of calories from people's diet come from soybean oil!

High-temperature processing also denatures fragile proteins to make soy protein isolate and textured vegetable protein. It seems the biggest problem with soy comes in its overuse in most heavily processed foods, isolated from the innocent G–d given soybean (non-GMO and all) it once was.

THE CONTROVERSY

Other controversial aspects of soy can be broken down into these categories:

1. Anti-nutrients
2. Isoflavone – phytoestrogens
3. Genetically Modified Organisms (GMO's)

1. Anti-Nutrients

We talked about phytic acid and the ability of fermentation to reduce some of those issues with grains. Phytates may obstruct the absorption of minerals like copper, iron, calcium, magnesium, and zinc in the intestinal tract. The phytates in soy actually enhance the concentration of genistein.

Unfermented soy contributes enzyme inhibitors, which interfere with the process of digestive enzymes, such as amylase lipase and protease, from being secreted in the digestive tract to help break down the soy and free nutrients after it is eaten. Because of this, the soybean carbohydrates and proteins are not completely digested. As a result, your bacteria try to break down the components of the food in the gut, causing bloating and other symptoms.

Could it be that fermented soy will solve most of these problems?

In some cases, yes. The process also allows the beneficial properties, like probiotics, to become available to your digestive system, enhancing nutrient absorption and contributing a plethora of healthy bacteria to the gut, which boosts your immunity. Fermented soy also shows properties including inhibiting cancer, osteoporosis, and other cardiovascular disease. Unlike the case with grain, only fermented soy neutralizes the phytic acid, but sprouting concentrates it. The forms of miso, tempeh, and natto are types of fermented soy:

o **Natto** is a form of soybeans fermented with the Mitoku natto spores and, in the Japanese diet, most often eaten with breakfast. It contains nattokinase, which acts as a potent blood thinner similar to taking an aspirin. Natto has one of the highest sources of vitamin k2, vital in fertility, with a beneficial probiotic called bacillus subtilis and a good source of protein. You may have to acquire a taste for the sticky texture, strong cheese-like flavor, and powerful smell.

o **Tempeh** is a fermented soybean pressed into a cake, similar to a veggie burger, or crumbled like taco meat. Tempeh is used as a meat substitute because of its firm texture and nutty, mushroom-like flavor.

o **Miso**, a thick, soybean paste fermented with koji bacteria, is high in protein and other vitamins and mineral. Miso tastes salty and has a buttery texture (commonly used in dashi and miso soups). Some also use miso to pickle vegetables and meats or as an added flavor to sauces and dressings.

o **Soy sauce** originated in China. Traditionally, the process entails soybeans made into a paste, combined with a roasted grain and fermented with aspergillus bacteria, which are pressed, producing the liquid soy sauce. Be careful when choosing a soy sauce on the market today because it may be made artificially using a chemical process.

o **Tamari**, produced in Japan, contains little or no wheat. Wheat-free tamari can be used by people with gluten intolerance. It was the first Japanese soy sauce, which closely resembles the soy sauce originally introduced to Japan from China. Technically, this is the liquid that runs off miso as it matures.

2. Soy Isoflavones

The soybean's isoflavones are a phytoestrogen necessary for the body. They are also found in beans and other legumes, including chickpeas and peanuts, and are closely related to the antioxidant flavonoid found in other plants like the cocoa bean. People seem to have a love-hate relationship with these polyphenol compounds. Specifically, soybeans have the glycosides genistein and daidzein, isoflavones that are shown to prevent cancer, but in large, processed amounts, can be cancer-promoting under specific circumstances.

3. GMO (Genetically Modified Organism)

About 80 percent or more of soy grown in the United States is genetically modified (see GMO in chapter 7). To avoid purchasing soy with GMOs, buy certified organic, which cannot contain GMOs by definition, or products that say, non-GMO on the label.

Limiting your intake of heavily processed food in general also helps minimize your isolated soy intake, a practice we are aiming to accomplish by living a real life with a real-food diet for other more healthful reasons, too.

SOY AND YOUR THYROID

Many people, especially women, suffer from low thyroid activity in America. Goitrogens are a compound found in soy and many other foods like cruciferous veggies (kale, cauliflower, broccoli, and cabbage) that may affect thyroid function. Some argue goitrogens alone slow down thyroid function by blocking the production of thyroid hormones, causing goiter formation and, eventually, causing thyroid cancer. But there are usually many other mechanisms at play causing those effects, such as iodine deficiency, the immune system, and metabolic problems in the liver.[115]

Fermentation does not necessarily help alleviate the effects of goitrogens, as the process actually frees the isoflavones (goitrogens) from their conjoined sugars and permits greater absorption. To help alleviate some effects of consuming goitrogens with soy, eat a diet rich in other iodine-rich foods.

THE ALLERGY

Soy is one of the most common food allergies, along with: wheat, cow's milk, hen's eggs, fish, crustacean shellfish (including shrimp, prawns, lobster, and crab); tree nuts (including cashews, almonds, walnuts, pecans, pistachios, Brazil nuts, hazelnuts, and chestnuts), and peanuts.

If you choose to incorporate more soy into your diet, take note of an allergic reaction such as breathing problems or skin rashes and symptoms triggered from a soy intolerance, such as nausea, vomiting, diarrhea, bloating, and constipation.

Cooking with Soy

Because raw soybeans (including the immature green form) are toxic, they should be cooked with "wet" heat to destroy the trypsin inhibitors (serine protease inhibitors).

- Soybeans can be cooked and eaten as is or used to make tofu and other fermented foods. The different forms can be added to pastas, salads, patties, and grilled, too.
- Mix sprouted soybeans into salads or use as toppings for sandwiches.
- Frozen edamame is simple to prepare and makes a great snack or appetizer. Just add the soybean pods to slightly salted water and boil for approximately ten minutes.
- Add soybeans to vegetable stews and soups.

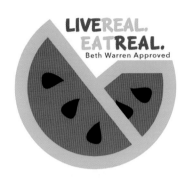

Because the research is double-sided, the take home message is to eat whole soy in moderation, rotated amongst other high-quality protein sources, and balanced amongst other whole food groups. The types of soy with the most benefits are the fermented products like tempeh, miso, and annatto. Take caution when consuming the more processed soy varieties such as soy milk, soy flour, and ingredients including soy protein isolates and soy lecithin, in large amounts, as they are found in most packaged goods. Lucky for you, that is the goal of choosing to live a real life with real food!

Enjoying soy foods, like tofu, edamame, and other good-quality proteins—in the context of eating other whole foods and rotating your food choices frequently—will ensure you are taking advantage of the benefits of soy without overdoing the load on your system. To avoid potential negative effects of goitrogens, simply consume soy in the context of an iodine-rich diet, by including foods like fish in your meal plan. Eating small amounts of these foods will provide the cancer-protective effects of components of soy, like genistein, without causing other potential problems.

LIVING A REAL LIFE WITH REAL FOOD

"Whoever conducts himself in the ways we have set forth,
I will guarantee that he will not get sick throughout his
life. . . . He will not need a doctor and his body will be in
perfect shape and remain healthy all his life."

Mishneh Torah, Hilchot De'ot 4:20

CHAPTER 9

EATING OUT AND INTO THE UNKNOWN WORLD OF REAL FOOD

"And Abraham went quickly into the tent to Sarah and said,
'Quick! Three seahs of fine flour! Knead it, and make cakes.'
And Abraham ran to the herd and took a calf, tender and
good, and gave it to a young man, who prepared it quickly.
Then he took curds and milk and the calf that he had prepared,
and set it before them. And he stood by them under the tree
while they ate."

—*Genesis 18:6-8*

Bang, Clang, Plop, Crash! Can you guess where I am?

Here's another hint: white subway-tile walls, ceramic floors, stainless steel pots and pans . . . need more?

Picture this: chefs cooking, aprons flying, vegetables chopping, food sizzling, and the aroma of exotic flavor in the air.

I am in a restaurant kitchen and studies show that many of you are nearby, too. The USDA reported that we eat 29 percent of our meals away from home, accounting for up to 44 percent of our food budgets, creeping up to 53 percent in the next few years, according to the National Restaurant Association. I would be remiss not to adequately address eating out in the unknown real world of temptation.

EATING OUT, THE DEFINITION

I define *eating out* as eating food outside your home, typically in a social setting. The foods may be prepared by someone at a restaurant, in a friend's home, or at gatherings such as weddings, holiday meals, birthday parties, or other events.

AT A FRIEND OR RELATIVE'S GATHERING

In the Jewish Community, social events are commonplace and food is tantalizingly featured. From extravagant occasions to routine Sabbath Friday night and Saturday lunch meals, the temptation to bite off more than you can chew at an event is part of our real world.

What happens when an invitation comes for you in the mail? You may read the details of the event and feel anxious, thinking, "How will I navigate the Food Unknown?" Fear not. With these real-food, real-world tips, you can combat any meal at a social gathering.

PLAN AHEAD

The golden rule responsible for a successful night spent eating out is planning. The day of, be sure to maintain your meal and snack times, eating the most fiber and protein-rich food combinations you have in your repertoire (See Meal Plans). Your goal is to make your stomach feel as full and satisfied as possible so you can fuel your mind to resist food temptations out of the home. Starving before you leave (a state of hunger many people strive for before going out because they want to fit in a certain dress or think they would gain the permission to overeat at the event) is setting yourself up for failure. Our brain needs sugar to function. If you don't eat for hours before the event, you won't be thinking efficiently.

Another important reason to choose nutrient-dense foods the day of the event is to leave a little wiggle room to indulge in one preplanned treat. If you know the typical food and dessert display at your destination, then plan out your plate beforehand. Know yourself: if you cannot resist your sister's apple cobbler, then tell yourself coming into the dinner that you will eat and enjoy one piece. This way, you will not see all the tempting sweets and lose control after inevitably tasting one bite. On the flipside, if you go into the event thinking *I will not touch a treat*, but you do have a taste, all bets are off. Psychologically, the pressure of restriction triggers your mind to think, "If I took one bite, I may as well eat everything." Be real with yourself first before you can be real about food.

Once hunger is taken out of the equation, we combat the psychological urges involved with social eating. Countless times, I have heard my patients report, "Beth, I didn't know why I was eating; I wasn't even hungry!" Reality is that most of the time you are eating for other reasons than hunger and it is important to identify what that reason is. It could be you are eating because:

1. Everyone else is eating.
2. The food is in front of you.

3. Someone is pressuring you to eat, "Why are you not eating?" "Are you on a diet?" "Please taste my dessert!"
4. You are feeling famished.
5. You are bored.
6. You forbid yourself from having any foods, but after eating one, you lose all self-control.
7. It just tastes *so* good. Period.
8. You think you probably won't see food like this again.
9. You have no idea how, but your hand is grazing the cookie plate multiple times.

Any of these sound familiar? Take a time-out before reaching the food and ask yourself, "Am I really hungry? Why do I want to eat this food?" If the answer sounds like one of the above excuses, do yourself a huge favor and follow some of these tips. I introduced them at one of my Lose Weight, Win Money, Gain Health challenges. At first, I was met with skepticism. Then, the women realized that their overeating at events had less to do with the food and more to do with a loss of taking control in social settings. Here are the non-food tips they tried (adapted from Connie Bennett, author of the bestselling books *Sugar Shock* and *Beyond Sugar Shock*, wrote in a Huffington Post article[116]):

See Yourself the Morning After
To prevent one Shabbat of overeating and "sinning" (i.e., overindulging on sweets, carbs, and high-fat foods) is to pretend that you're talking to a friend or loved one the next day and openly sharing what happened at your feast. What would you say to this person? Would you be embarrassed? Would you be too mortified to tell her or him that you lost control? My clients find that having to honestly dish the dirt to a loved one can prevent them from overeating. Or talk to yourself in the mirror—the mind–body connection is powerful!

Do the Timed Breath, Blow-Out Technique
When you're sitting around your friend's meal and sweets, carbs, or other rich foods "call out" to you, let your watch help you to slow

down. Before you shove that second (or even first) serving of candy into your mouth:

- Check the time on your watch. (If you don't wear one, ask someone else.)
- Then, whatever time it is, take that number of breaths—but do so slowly, deliberately and confidently, breathing in and out slowly. So, let's say it's 9 a.m. That means you'll slowly, consciously take nine deep breaths in and nine breaths out.
- At the same time, visualize your breath whooshing or blowing away your craving up into the sky. (You can pretend that you're breathing away your cravings as if they are gentle clouds.) Expect that to occur. Now, watch your cravings go poof.
- If you're still tempted and are close to pigging out, repeat the whole procedure again. (You'll take another nine breaths.)
- If that still doesn't work and your cravings are really strong, then you can really buckle up. Take nine breaths nine times. (If it were 3 p.m., then you'd do three breaths three times, etc.)

Take Gratitude Breaks

Before you grab an extra helping, take a Gratitude Break. Go to a corner in your friend or family member's home (or your home) and think about the meaning behind Shabbat. Then, before you put any more food into your mouth, first think about twenty things for which you love Shabbat. (If you can, write them down before Shabbat and read them aloud if you're home.)

Give a Hug and a Compliment and Switch Your Focus

At Shabbat or another event, one of the best ways to quit focusing on food and sweets is to think about someone else. Find a guest or two (someone you don't know that well or even your least favorite relative) and give that person your undivided attention. If you can, find out from your host or hostess which of your relatives or loved ones is having the hardest time. Then, go over to that person, catch up, ask questions, and then listen carefully. Make sure to give this person your support, encouragement, validation, understanding, warmth, compassion, and love. When you're giving to another like this, your heart will open up and you'll be filled with warm, fuzzy, good feelings rather than food.

Say a Prayer . . . Again and Again

When those rich, sugar-filled junk foods and drinks are tempting you, pray to G–d to help you resist (silently) each time you're about to put a bite of food in your mouth. Then, if that doesn't work, thank the farmers who brought you the various elements of the meal. Next, silently thank the companies that may have been involved. And if you need to go further, give gratitude to G–d for rain, your house plant, or whatever catches your attention. Religious people have fun with this little trick and find that it helps to lead to weight loss. Essentially, all this thanking takes time. So delving deeply into gratitude like this can slow you down and help keep you from overeating.

Have Fun after the Feast

Soon after the evening begins, organize some kind of fun group activity. You could all go for a walk in the neighborhood, play a game of cards, or maybe you could all sing some pizmonim, or Jewish psalms. Just find an activity that you can involve the most guests in enjoying. You will then look forward to your big game or walk or whatever activity you organize and you'll become less interested in pigging out on all the sweets and overeating the foods offered during your meal.

Tell a Joke

As we all know, it's darn difficult to eat or overeat when you're laughing. So if you're clamoring after sweets or quickie carbs, tell a joke. In other words, figure out a way to make yourself laugh. You'll not only keep yourself from overeating, but you may get the whole table laughing so hard that they become less interested in their meal. (If you like, you could study some joke books in advance to have some good comedy material.)

Keep Close Track

Make a promise to your best friend or loved one (or, for now, *me*) to write down every single bite that you consume on Shabbat afterward.

The idea of having to share your food list with someone else is quite intimidating and just keeping a what-I-ate-at-Shabbat list can prevent pigging out.

When in Doubt, B.Y.O.F.

The following tip is for people with special sensitivities. If you find it hard to keep control over the holidays or if you are allergic to gluten, meat, dairy, or other substances, you may want to Bring Your Own Food (B.Y.O.F.). For instance, when I was in Israel for a year, I always brought my own dessert to my host's house so I could be sure I liked one part of the meal. Likewise, I currently try to accommodate my guests with their taste preferences if they have food allergies and other personal health issues. If you have not yet trained your relatives and friends, then you may wish to bring some foods that will enable you to stay on track.

AT A RESTAURANT

BEFORE YOU LEAVE

Your first choice in selecting a restaurant should be one with a variety of foods on the menu. In advance, review the restaurant's menu online, ask them to fax or email you a copy, or discuss some choices over the phone with the hostess so you can make your meal decisions before you get there.

It is better to distinguish what kind of meal you are looking for, decide on one, and eat it—not avoid it. Think about what foods you are craving: pasta, fish, something salty or sweet? Does the restaurant have the one dish you absolutely love and cannot resist? Your goal is not to be tempted by other items on the menu by planning your choice ahead of time. Some patients of mine do well with recording their calorie counts throughout the day and focus on not going over on their caloric load for the day at their restaurant meal; however, I like to utilize the day to have more nutrient-dense foods to fully fuel and satisfy yourself coming into the dinner so, overall, you will take in fewer calories for the day.

A good idea is to set a reservation, decreasing the likelihood of getting too hungry or resorting to drinks at the bar while waiting in line for a table. Ask them to seat your party at a table away from the kitchen so you are neither tempted visually or aromatically by the more caloric dishes.

While speaking with the restaurant staff, feel free to ask how they usually prepare their meals. Are most of the dishes fried, baked, or steamed? Do they accommodate substitutions on the menu?

It is critical that one to two hours before leaving the house, you eat a small, nutrient-dense snack. Snacks should consist of foods that are high in fiber and protein, such as an apple with one tablespoon of natural peanut butter. If you are running short on time, a simple apple or one ounce of nuts, unsalted, is sufficient. If you miss this step, you are more likely to eat the "table foods," like bread and butter, that wait innocently with the words EAT ME stamped onto the tablecloth.

If your restaurant allows, bring your own whole-wheat melba toast, a homemade dressing, or any other healthy choices they may not offer. It is always better to be over-prepared. Most kosher restaurants, however, do not allow you to bring outside food into the restaurant, so be sure to study their meal options as best you can beforehand and plan your choices accordingly.

SITTING AT YOUR TABLE

You can start the night off right by politely requesting the waiter take back the free items. I'm aware of how difficult this may be, but my patients have proven that this one step paves the way for a successful night of healthy, guilt-free eating. Skipping the bread and butter will easily help you shave 200 to 300 calories off your meal.

If you must have the bread on the table because your guest insists (rationalization or truth), ask for whole wheat and eat it plain. If you need a spread, ask for a lower-calorie alternative to butter or have extra virgin olive oil instead.

The second you sit at the table and before you begin to feel overwhelmed, start sipping water. Drinking may help ward off some of what feels like the urge to eat, so you can be sure what you are experiencing is not thirst. Also, we sometimes feel the need to be doing something with our hands and mouth in a social setting and having a cup of water in hand may be enough. Finally, do yourself a favor and remove any dessert or specials menu displayed on the table to decrease the temptation of ordering from them.

HOW TO ORDER

The moment has come and you are ready to order your meal. Keep in mind: this is not a time to be polite. I give you permission to be the first to order so you will not tempted by the dishes ordered by the rest of your party. How many times have we heard or told ourselves after making our choice of what to eat, "Oh, that sounds good, maybe I'll try that one"?

Additionally, if your server comes, but you are not ready to order, you do not have to make a quick decision you may regret. At the same time, if you singled out your choice and are ready to order, call the waiter over as quickly as possible and hand back the menu as fast and final as submitting your tax returns by the deadline. Signed, sealed, delivered, and done.

Often times, it is necessary to encourage my patients to ask questions or make special requests when ordering food. I want you to gain the confidence to ask for what you want. No vegetables listed? You want to switch a bread or pasta to whole wheat? Ask for substitutions! Restaurants are in business to serve. You should be able to request a dish you want. The worst that can happen is they say no. Getting in the habit of choosing the food you want to eat instead of the menu items choosing you is a sign you are living a real life with real food. You, not the food, are in charge of *you*.

You can also ask about the portions sizes of the dishes. At times, a side dish or an appetizer with a salad makes a great meal if the other options are too big. A study published in the *Journal of Consumer Research* showed that eating off a smaller plate, or an appetizer-sized meal, would result in you eating 9 to 31 percent less than if you ate off a larger plate.[117]

When deciding on a dish, take note of which foods have cheeses, sour creams, gravies, and special sauces. Ideally, you should not order these additional items or, if you need or want them, you should ask for them on the side. These ingredients are usually what make the meal go from controlled to excessive, oftentimes because of salt, calories, and sugar. If you want the flavor of the sauces, dip your fork, not the actual food, in the condiment and spread over your food. A teaspoon in total is a good rule of thumb for a measurement of condiments per meal. "Extras" also include preparation methods that add oil, butter, and sugar; request these not be added to your plate.

I have witnessed a gourmet pizza maker paintbrush olive oil onto the crust at his restaurant just before serving and an ice cream shop server squirting chocolate syrup into an already chocolate-flavored milk shake. These are additions that are unnecessary to both flavor and calories. Most people I encounter are not aware of these extras. I bet that if you ask them not to add anything like oil, syrup, and sugar, you will hardly notice the change in taste, flavor, and satisfaction—but your body will notice the change in calories and will thank you.

Take the opportunity to be the painter you always wanted to be and design your dish to be as colorful as a rainbow. Typically, a plate filled with bland colors like brown, beige, white, or pale yellow is an indication that you are having a high-calorie, high-fat, heavily starched meal. A colorful palette also helps with visual stimulation and enjoyment of your meal, which helps you feel satisfied and happy after eating.

If your situation allows, order one course at a time. We have a habit to order with our eyes, not our bellies. After eating an appetizer and waiting twenty minutes for the main course, you may honestly not be hungry. When your meal finally comes, it's harder to deny its passage into your body. If you wait to order, take the twenty minutes to enjoy your company and allow your belly to communicate with your mind that you are full and satisfied (See chapter 3).

APPETIZERS

If you want to start the meal off on a positive note, foods including vegetables and fruits are good choices as long as they are not dipped, fried, or breaded, but rather steamed. Take note of the appetizers as you search the main dish options because an appetizer and a salad make a great, well-portioned meal.

SOUPS AND SALADS

These two items serve as a meal in and of themselves. Starting your meal with a broth-based soup, like a simple vegetable soup, versus creamier textures is proven to help save calories in your complete meal. However, semi-creamy mushroom and barley, split pea, and lentil soups are healthier options because they are packed with fiber that will help you feel fuller and more satisfied throughout your meal.

Before you think you can never go wrong with vegetables, think again. A lot of hidden calories hide in a restaurant's salad bar. Skip over the oily croutons, pasta or potato salads, and stick with typical choices of carrots, peppers, tomatoes, and cucumbers. Add nuts, garbanzo, kidney, and black beans for additional sources of protein and true healthy colors. Experiment with different dark green flavors, textures, and nutrients such as spinach leaves, kale, and arugula . . . or mix them together!

Dressings are a potential salad bar pitfall but can still be enjoyed. The best option is a simple lemon juice and olive oil dressing or add red wine or balsamic vinegar. Aside from being a real-food option, you use less of liquid-based dressings than creamy ones to cover the entire salad (about

4 tablespoons). Creamy dressings are conserved to 2 tablespoons. Ask yourself, "Which option will give me more bang for my health buck?" Trust me, the lemon-and-olive-oil option is more satisfying to stomach, mind, and body.

ENTRÉE

Finally, you are ready to choose your entrée. Believe it or not, the most nervewracking part of your meal choice is actually the simplest to decipher. Avoid the words: *buttery, breaded, buttered, fried, pan-fried, creamed, scalloped, au gratin,* and *à la mode.* Find the words: *grilled, baked, steamed, boiled, poached, stir-fried, roasted,* and *blackened.* Avoid heavy sauces made with ingredients including milk, cheese, mayonnaise, or white-based colors. Instead choose a red-colored marinara or tomato-based sauces as a general indication that the dish is a healthier option. Either way, ask for your sauce on the side or replace with other herbs and spices for added flavor. At the very least, ask for the chef to go light on your sauce.

Your choice of proteins is another area where you can choose to be healthier. The fatty and lean meats are important to recognize:

o **Fish:** all fairly lean or contain healthy fat.
o **Chicken:** fairly lean, especially when skin and fat is removed. White is leaner than dark meat, but not by too many calories. The same rules apply to **turkey** and **duck**.
o **Ground beef products** (in order of most to least fat): ground beef, ground chuck, ground round. Eye of round and roasts are leaner, while steaks and ribs have more fat.
o If you are ordering a **prime rib** or **roast**, request the leaner center or inner cut.

Keep in mind the serving size of meat is 3 to 4 ounces. If your plate gets served to you with the steak covering the entire area, make sure to immediately request to package half to take home.

If you are vegetarian or choose a vegetarian option, tread cautiously. The menu options are not always healthier and the same tips apply.

Side Dishes

You have an opportunity to turn the health tides of your entire meal with the side dishes. I often make my own requests if there are not healthier options. Asking for a side of vegetables is an accommodation most restaurants can make. Try not to allow any other thoughts of unhealthier sides creep into your mind. If a meal comes with two side options, even better. Request one cooked option like steamed, stewed, or broiled broccoli and a raw vegetable, like salad, to keep it flavorful. Be careful with the mayonnaise-based sides, such as coleslaw and potato salad, as these can be high in calories.

The retort "But the dish came with fries" is no excuse to succumb to the french fries, fried potato, hash browns, chips, or other fatty food temptation. There is always a better option like a small baked, broiled, or roasted potato with no added creams, sauces, oils, or butters—so choose wisely! If you need added flavor, request salsa, chives, pepper, or veggies to mix with the potato. If veggies are simply not an option, try a fruit salad.

Dessert

As dinner winds down, you pray, "Please don't ask if I want dessert!" Alas, the question becomes reality and now you have to answer. Ideally, you and everyone in your party decline the invitation. If they decide to order and you feel uncomfortable not ordering (a feeling of confidence I encourage you to practice!), request a hot tea or coffee. If you need food, fresh fruit as dessert is always the best option—with no added sauces or whipped cream. Sorbets or frozen yogurts are better than ice cream; however, be sure to keep your serving size to 4 ounces and be mindful of sugar content.

You are allowed to indulge from time to time. But the worst that can happen is you feel so deprived that you eat one cookie and it becomes ten cookies and is accompanied by a hopeless feeling of guilt. A sign on my office door puts it clearly: KEEP CALM AND HAVE A CUPCAKE! "Keep Calm" being the important point.

A prime example of how one indulgence can catapult into a larger problem takes place during the holiday season. Holiday weight gain is not a reflection on the holiday itself, but the result of one indulgent night eating out leading to two, three, and so on. Indulging does not have to become a habit. Tomorrow is a new day and it is crucial you pick yourself up and say you will do better next time. My way of compensating for indulgences is waking up the next morning, welcoming the fresh start, drinking a lot of water, and being sure to fit in an intense workout—no matter what was already scheduled on my calendar for the day.

I went to a gourmet pizza shop to write a restaurant review one evening. I inquired about their chocolate pizza, which some of my patients asked me about. While I had not ordered it, to my surprise, the chocolate pizza dessert was in my stack of take-out boxes. (I wonder who did that?) The description alone and the manager's warning on its high-calorie content was reason enough to steer clear. Being a chocolate lover, there was no way to avoid it while it was sitting in front of me. One bite and I was, deliciously, in heaven. I had not felt the urge to consume anything this caloric in a long time, but boy, was this worth it! If there were ever a way to treat myself, this chocolate pizza was it. The night ended, but my will power did not. The next day, I was back in charge of my food choices.

A healthier way to deal with an indulgence is purchasing any dessert you choose with a group of friends, and as soon as the dish hits your table, have everyone rush to grab *one* spoonful. If not, you'll end up eating the whole thing, no matter how strong your will power is . . . dessert can be *that* delicious.

When it comes to a Shabbat or any gathering for that matter, focus on keeping portions smaller, not bigger. Oversizing (unless it is with veggies) is *not* okay. So go for tiny portions without the guilt. For example, opt for one small "pick me up" dark chocolate dessert as opposed to a huge piece of cake.

REAL EATING

You spot your dish from a mile away. Steam is emitting from the tantalizing meal about to be displayed before you. After all the effort you put into choosing your ideal real-food dish, you feel like clapping in excitement and anticipation, but you think twice when you realize there are eyes on you. That's okay. You are having a relationship with your food and the feeling is mutual. Now that you have your meal, take the time to enjoy it, literally. Between each bite, put your fork down, chew, sip water, and enjoy the conversations of your companion(s).

When deciding on the first bite, the same rules of eating at home apply: crunch on your veggies first, then protein, and finally, the starch. Eat the amount you typically would at home, on your comforting nine-inch plate. Mid-way through your meal, ask yourself, "Am I hungry?" and answer honestly. If not, request the server pack your food to take home. If your meal setting does not allow for you to wave the waiter over, put a napkin over your dish—out of sight out of mind.

While your company is finishing their food, keep your hands busy: drink a beverage, hold hands with your date, or just sit on them! If you need to, excuse yourself. Use the restroom and grab an after-dinner mint early to suck on it or chew gum.

I fully endorse eating out as part of your real life. Ideally, you should be eating home with foods prepared by you as often as possible. But, the occasional restaurant indulgence is warranted and should be enjoyed!

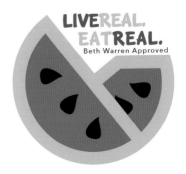

LIVE REAL.
EAT REAL.
Beth Warren Approved

Indulgences can still be smart choices and should be centered on your path toward better health. The important point to keep in mind is that there is always a better choice. If you are only given options A or B, you need to believe you have the power to create option C. Feel confident in requesting foods you want and how they should be prepared and, of course, enjoy your time out with friends and loved ones. If the restaurant was able to accommodate your healthier requests, be sure to give them positive feedback and note the name of the restaurant for your next night out.

If you steer off your healthier path, you should know, deep inside your mind and body, that tomorrow is a new day to regain control over your foods. Take comfort knowing that you made the best choices you could make and asked the best questions you could ask. Confidence in knowing that you can incorporate real foods into your real life, even if outside the home, is an important hurdle to overcome.

These tips for eating out can be applied to Sabbath and holiday meals as well. The goal is to try to make these days fit into your real-food diet by making it like any other day: try to wake up at the same time everyday, eat your real-food snacks at the right times, create your "plate" at meal times, and be sure to eat a real-food snack before you go out to eat. If you want to indulge in a dessert, go for a dark chocolate treat (about 1 oz) or 6 dark chocolate covered nuts or one fruit serving, and try to choose one time of day to have it, either with the dinner or lunch meals, but not both. (I prefer lunchtime since you may have more control over what you eat than the nighttime.) Remember, delay, delay, delay . . . you may not want a dessert if you avoided the impulse to eat.

Eating out with real food in your real life gets my Kosher Seal of Approval.

CHAPTER 10

SUPERMARKET SWEEP

"When the famine had spread over the whole country, Joseph opened all the storehouses and sold grain to the Egyptians, for the famine was severe throughout Egypt. And all the world came to Egypt to buy grain from Joseph, because the famine was severe everywhere."

—*Genesis, 41:56*

I fondly recall memories from childhood of a favorite television game show called *Supermarket Sweep*. Two challengers were given one shopping wagon and one minute and thirty seconds on the clock to fill it with the highest valued products they could find. I anxiously watched the contestants fly through the aisles, throwing items like turkey and cuts of meat haphazardly into their carts. I longed to know exactly which items were strategically higher valued and how someone could possibly finish supermarket shopping in a minute and a half. Today, my goal is practically the same: to know which high-quality items to throw into my cart for better health in the least amount of time.

Although the timer was part of the show's competition, the one minute and thirty seconds on the clock is closer to our supermarket shopping reality. Amongst our real lives of tending to children, spouses, friends, work, and other daily tasks, we may not have the time to spend strolling through the aisles to find real food to buy. If only it can be like the biblical times of Joseph—the Bible describes the first reference to a supermarket. During the great famine, Joseph foresaw through Pharaoh's dreams that there would be seven years of plenty. Joseph had the idea, and was put in charge of collecting food and building storage houses. Come the time of the seven years of famine, people flocked to the storage houses (or what I like to call the first supermarket) and bought grains. The process was simple: go in and buy grains in a place that stored only grains, and one left with only grains.

Nowadays, our stores are larger and filled with items other than "what we really need." From prepared foods to household products and toiletries, even magazines and DVDs, we are not only shorter on time, but need to make a bigger effort to find the products we want for better health. On top of everything, we have the manipulation of the supermarket design persuading us to buy foods we do not need, and we often leave the store without the products we do need.

How can we quickly sift through the poor-quality foods and find the real ones in these vast supermarkets? In this chapter, I will break down the purchasing guidelines of packaged real foods so you can enjoy them in your busy real life.

THE INNOVATIONS

As much as you would like to think that the goal of a supermarket is to help you on your path to better health, think again. The goal of a supermarket is to sell its products. Some products need more marketing strategies to get you to want to buy it. The supermarket starts to influence your decision making the second you walk through the door. Whole Foods Market® is known for incorporating many strategies to increase your shopping experience from the get-go. They play familiar music that makes you nostalgic and allows you to "feel good," so you are inclined to buy more. They handwrite their signs with their two staffed artists for an appealing and homey look and feel to the store. The products they sell are of a higher quality so you spend more on them. The fruits and vegetable display is arranged by color so it is aesthetically pleasing. You are hit with aromatics of fresh, prepared foods organized throughout the store. Seemingly countless employees are on duty, meeting your every need, question, or desire. Each of your senses is activated in a relaxing, attractive, and enticing way, priming you to buy more.

As much as they want us to believe otherwise, you do not have to walk into a Whole Foods® to find quality food. On the other end of the spectrum is Wal-Mart®, and somewhere in the middle are stores like Safeway. Because of our consumer behavior, many of these stores carry quality foods at a lower price than Whole Foods® or even Trader Joe's®, but most likely carry more foods that are lower quality to keep their price points low and cater to a different clientele. The more you change your buying behavior, the more all stores will reflect a healthier inventory.

One of the best ways a supermarket makes a profit with lower margins is with their own supermarket brand. From ShopRite® to Trader Joe's® and, more recently, Whole Foods® with their 365 Everyday Value® brand, some supermarkets make their own line of food products. If they are comparable to other quality products you are buying, then take advantage of the lower price point and purchase them. Our goal is to buy quality food, not a certain brand or the more expensive option.

One suggestion you may have heard for finding healthy foods in a supermarket setting is to shop the perimeter of the store for the best choices. While these areas usually have excellent options of fresh foods like fruits and vegetables, the innovative designs introduced to some markets may have some interesting kosher, real-food finds within the aisles, as well.

START SMALL

● ●

Frequently, I run supermarket tours to help guide consumers on how to shop for real food in places like Dean's Natural Market® in New Jersey. I like to conduct them in a smaller market committed to quality foods. As you begin to incorporate real foods into your real life, I recommend you follow suit and start in a small specialty market committed to real food choices. It is best to see all the options available, in a less overwhelming way and without so many unwanted choices. Although these settings have better-quality options most of the time, you still need to have on your investigative hats to find the best products that are both better for your health and are worth the extra penny (see Tips).

Health food co-ops are another good choice if they are available in your area; they typically have sales on their products, which make them a more affordable venue. You can also try shopping at your local farmers' markets. Not only will you get better quality, local foods, you will "shake the hand that feeds you," as Michael Pollan writes in his book, *In Defense of Food: An Eater's Manifesto.* You cannot beat education from the mouth of the source that is providing you with G–d's fresh food. Farmers' markets also allow for a pleasurable shopping experience, which encourages you to buy fresh, local produce, pastured eggs, and other new ingredients with which you can experiment.

Once you find the brands you like and become educated on the pricing and good health choices, you can spread your wings to cover larger supermarkets with better-quality food from places such as Wegman's®, Whole Foods®, and Trader Joe's®. To begin in these larger supermarkets will be overwhelming at first, so start small, feel confident, and add additional supermarkets as you become more comfortable shopping for real food.

WALKING THROUGH THE DOOR

The first things you face upon entering a supermarket are two sections: the decompression zone and fresh fruits and vegetables. While the produce section speaks for itself, the decompression zone is meant to "prime" you by slowing you down to take in your surroundings. Wal-Mart® is known for using "greeters" for this priming purpose. Priming applies to repeat customers, as well, so supermarkets are often changing what you see first, such as refreshing the magazine stands or bulk-bargains, to make a new experience for you at every visit.

The fruits and vegetables section hits you first for many reasons. Think about it: if you add in fresh fruits and veggies, would you feel as guilty tossing in the mac and cheese or chocolate bars? No, because you balanced it with the fresh produce you picked up earlier.

The standard supermarket is designed to promote consumption of high-sugar and high-preservative foods because those have high margins and maximize profit. These supermarkets do not have to designate more than five hundred square feet for fresh produce, in an average ten thousand square-foot space.

The aisle display is also planned. Products are lined up horizontally and displayed in a way where the color pops. Brown boxes of chocolate cake mixes will be lined up next to yellow cake mixes for contrasts in color. Aside from being aesthetically pleasing, the placement allows consumers to sense a difference in flavor (chocolate versus fudge) instead of overlooking the different items and seeing them both as the same flavor if they were next to each other.

The design of the supermarket is also meant to keep you in there for a longer time. The more time spent inside, the more you are presumed to buy. It is quite the opposite of our real-life plan to quickly get in and out. They intentionally make it more difficult for you to find the products you need by placing items they want you to buy along the way. This can explain why you only find pharmacies and staple products like milk and eggs in the back of the store.

In the end, there is a reason why you are so confused about what products to buy and why you may leave the supermarket without the products you wanted—and with a slew of others you did not intend to buy. It's not only you; it is emphatically the odds of the grocery store strategic plans working against you.

When it comes down to it, a supermarket design is a science, created to make you spend more on marketed brand products and buy more processed foods. It's not that supermarkets don't want you to buy fruits and vegetables. On the contrary, there is a greater risk of loss here because they can spoil. But fruits' and vegetables' wholesomeness sells themselves. They do not need to do any strategic manipulations to sell them. It is foods we do not need for better health that have to be marketed in order for us to feel like we have to have it. And let's face it: it works.

YOUR BUYER POWER

Interestingly, years ago supermarkets would place heavier items at the beginning of the shopping experience and lighter products at the end. The reason was practical: you would be less likely to crush the lighter items in your cart. However, today's design has shifted in the opposite direction because consumers are shopping differently. We are more often shopping the perimeters of the store, which means that we are putting lighter items, like fruits and vegetables, in the cart first. Health became a priority in our lives and our shopping strategy changed. As a result, the supermarket design changed. In the end, as much as we are victim to the strategic manipulations of a supermarket design trying to control what and how much we buy, we do have the power to change that same strategy by changing our shopping behaviors.

Never doubt your consumer power. If there is a product you want a supermarket to carry, ask for it! If there is something you like about the supermarket, including how they display products or what they carry, then verbalize positive feedback so they continue to please you. You *can* change how your supermarket is designed and the products carried. You have that power as a consumer: know it, believe it, and act on it!

NEVER GO HUNGRY

I used to visit my grandmother, Sarah (may she rest in peace), in Florida during the winter months. The first thing we did was go food shopping. I would often arrive close to the Sabbath, so our first stop was at a Syrian specialty store with easy-to-find Sabbath items, including fresh-made Syrian delicacies like Lahemb'ajeen and Kibbeh. Every year as we approached the store, she would say, "Don't ever come here hungry." I laughed at her humor. The store was known to be very expensive, and if you went in hungry, you were sure to buy more because of the enticing aromas and novelty products permeating the store. She couldn't have been more right! With that advice in mind, I give you my quick tips on supermarket shopping:

Top Rules on Supermarket Shopping

o   Never go into a supermarket hungry.
o   Always have a shopping list written down. *Written* ideally means hand-written. There are good apps on the smartphone today, but just like the food records, I find the old-fashioned pen and paper even more effective.
o   If you have a small order, only take a hand basket. If you need one or two products, then only buy what you can hold in your arms, without the aid of a basket. This is a foolproof method I use so I don't buy more than I intended.

o   Try to look up the sales in the circular or on a supermarket's website in advance so you are not enticed by surprising specials when you really did not need those items. Sometimes, if you had those few extra minutes to think about it, you would realize that, for example, you had a dozen paper towels waiting to be used in your storage closet. This also helps control buyer's remorse. There is little worse than buying things you did not need and feeling guilty afterwards.

o   Weigh the pros and cons about shopping in a large supermarket (with more options and bulk products) versus a smaller place that may be more costly but has features fewer manipulations to get you to buy more because there are fewer products in the store. I often find that if I go to a large supermarket, although the prices are cheaper and I am buying more for my money, I spend more than if I were to just pop into a local grocery that had the exact products I need—albeit more costly per item—and leaving without extra goodies. Ultimately, this is a decision you need to make based on your shopping budget, schedule, and household storage capacity.

o   Leave anyone who will influence what you buy at home! That means, husband, roommates, friends, kids, and others. Of course, I don't mean *every* time. But be aware of their manipulation in getting you to buy what they want. It's great to bring kids along, but make it a rule that they can only choose to buy real-food options and don't be afraid to tell them no. Resolving to only buy what is on the list is a good strategy to relay to whoever is accompanying you on your shopping experience.

o   Fill your cart with as many fresh foods as possible and real-food ingredients.

> o Put back products with more than two lines of ingredients or products that fill up their ingredient list with mostly unrecognizable chemicals.
> o Use apps like Fooducate for questionable items to make an informed, healthier decision.

WHAT TO LOOK FOR IN REAL-FOOD PRODUCTS

Some may say that if you are committed to eating a whole-food diet, then you cannot buy any packaged goods. While eating fresh is always best because you know what is going into the product and it is not laden with stabilizers and preservatives to keep a longer shelf life, sometimes it's not practical for your real life. If you cannot eat fresh, does that mean you need to abandon the whole, real-food diet? No! Because that would mean you are missing the second half to my philosophy—"for your real life." Eating real foods has to fit into *your real life*. If your real life is hectic, then I want to guide you on how to buy packaged goods that will allow you to hold true to your real-food goals, not abandon them. Remember, eating real food is a way of life, not a short-term diet. You should not feel guilty about needing some extra help from packaged goods now and again. At the same time, if you know you will need to buy packaged products, it is crucial you learn how to find the best-quality products (see Shopping List).

FOOD LABEL

The first place to start is with the food label. The consensus is that the food label is confusing and many parts of it are not applicable to the average person. At this time, food labels are currently undergoing research by the (FDA) in regards to making them easier to understand so you can make a more healthful choice. Most patients who come to see me do not understand what the current labels mean.

Now that we are fully aware of the negatives influenced upon us before we even walk into a supermarket, let us learn how to find the healthiest products on the shelves.

I love to challenge my patients with a food label when they come to see me. I always ask, "What do you look at first?" I have never found someone who does not look at the fat or calories first, so they are always surprised to see how I read a food label. I guarantee that if you look at the nutrition facts the way I do, and in my order, you will quickly sift through your shopping cart to find the real-food items, for

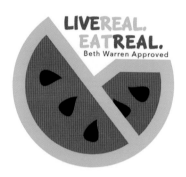

in the end, there are a lot of factors to consider when reading a food label. You should not write off a product because "it's fattening" or "has a lot of carb." The opposite is also true; you shouldn't choose a product because "it's only 100 calories." Instead, you should ask yourself these questions:

"Where are those carbs or fats coming from?"

"Are they from sources that will help or hurt my health?"

"Are these calories coming from quality sources that my body could use?"

"Are they the kinds that will help boost my metabolism or slow it down?"

There are a lot of variables to consider. Asking the right questions and looking for the right answers in your food label will help you find real food products.

Nutrition Facts

Serving Size 11 crisps (31g)

Amount Per Serving

Calories 120   Calories from fat 25

	%Daily Value
Total Fat 3g	5%
Saturated Fat 0g	0%
Trans Fat 0g	
Polyunsaturated Fat 1g	
Monounsaturated Fat 1.5g	
Cholesterol 0mg	0%
Sodium 180 mg	8%
Total Carbohydrate 22g	7%
Dietary Fiber 5g	18%
Insolube Fiber 3g	
Soluble Fiber 2g	
Sugars 2g	
Protein 3g	

Vitamin A	0%	Vitamin C	0%
Calcium	0%	Iron	2%

*Percent Daily Values are based on a 2,000 calorie diet. Your daily values may be higher or lower depending on your calorie needs:

	Calcium	2,000	2,500
Total Fat	Less than	65g	80g
Sat Fat	Less than	20g	25g
Cholesterol	Less than	300mg	300mg
Sodium	Less than	2,400mg	2,400mg
Total Carbohydrate		300g	375g
Dietary Fiber		25g	30g

Calories per gram:

Fat 9   •   Carboydrate 4   •   Protein 4

THE „REAL FOOD" APPROACH

TO NUTRITION FACTS UBELS

The first place I look is how many servings are in the food I am eating. This is a major factor in figuring out how much of what I am going to read below is in my serving.

HIGH FIBER IS REAL FOOD APPROVED

Fiber: Most highly processed foods are devoid of fiber (I could confidently assert this point until products like Kellogg's® Froot Loops® decided to fortify [add in an ingredient that does not naturally occur] with fiber, which does not make it a healthier food)! For the most part, better quality foods will have natural fiber. At a minimum, you want over two grams, but the more the better! I would love if you had over five grams of fiber in a product, especially cereals and starches. Fiber has a slew of health benefits and breaking them down by insoluble and soluble fiber is even better (see chapter 6).

LOW SUGAR IS REAL FOOD APPROVED

Sugar: Since I am in the realm of carbohydrates when I look at fiber (sugar and fiber are forms of carbohydrates and are included in the total carbohydrate count of a product), I look down into the sugar content. We want this number to be as low as possible. Ideally, your product should have less than ten grams of sugar. However, products like yogurt have natural sugar lactose, and may account for up to 12 grams of natural sugar. Although sugar is still sugar, the source does matter. You want to have as little added sugar in your diet as possible (the American Heart Association recommends sugar intake for adult women is 5 teaspoons [20 grams] of sugar per day; for adult men, it's 9 teaspoons [36 grams] daily; and for children, it's 3 teaspoons [12 grams] a day). The ingredient list will help you decipher if the sugar is added or natural.

QUALITY CALORIES IS REAL FOOD APPROVED

Calories: After the carbohydrate breakdown, I make my way up to the calorie count. Some people look here first. The reason why I do not is because the calorie count is an overall picture of the product. It does not specify where those calories are coming from. If you look here, you may miss the quality of your food. A 100-calorie snack pack will have less calories than 1 oz of almonds, but which is better quality for your health? If you followed my order, you would automatically see about 3.5 grams of fiber in almonds and zero in a 100-calorie snack pack and accurately, put the 100-calorie box back onto the shelf.

Fat: After noting how many calories are in the product, towards the right you will see how many calories are coming from fat. This number is not telling us much since we learned in chapter 4 that the kinds of fat matter. (In the amended nutrition facts label coming out, this line item may be taken away as it does not affect consumer behavior). Then, I make my way down to the fat content to see where these calories of fat are coming from. Again, this may be the first item you look at, but if you did, you would never eat healthy fats like avocado and will miss out on many good quality real foods that will help your weight-loss and better health goals. I skim over the total grams of fat and into the division of the specific grams of fat. For saturated fat, you want the number to ideally, be less than 1 gram. For **trans fat**, that number should be zero. The better quality foods may break down the fats further to include good fats like **monounsaturated and polyunsaturated fats**. If the grams of fat are coming from these good sources, you can be more confident that you are eating a better quality food. As much as the total fat is important, because fat does contribute the highest amounts of calories in your food, the quality of fats and their source matters.

LOW
SATURATED FAT
IS REAL FOOD
APPROVED

NO TRANS FAT
IS REAL FOOD
APPROVED

MORE
POLYUNSATURATED FAT
MONOUNSATURATED FAT
IS REAL FOOD
APPROVED

Sodium: After fat, I skip down to the sodium, which should be as low as possible. If you need to buy packaged prepared foods like soups,do not choose one over 250 mg of sodium. When you are going over 300 mg of sodium in a product, put it back. Most processed foods and packaged goods will have sodium, so it is hard to avoid. Aside from flavor, salt is the major ingredient in shelf-stability and freshness.This is a major consideration when you can choose to make fresh foods like soups and veggie burgers whenever possible: you control the sodium and only add for the purpose of flavor, if needed.

Cholesterol: It is important for this number to be low, but I am not as concerned as other fat levels. Saturated and trans fat, for example, are more likely to increase your blood cholesterol than the cholesterol in a real food, like eggs.

Protein: You want to aim for a high amount of quality protein. The amount depends on the type of product you are buying. For example, when buying a protein bar, you want the protein content to be above 10 grams (and less then 200 calories if it is a snack). These days, many highly processed foods may have some protein, which is why it is not the first item I look for on a food label, or you may be tricked into choosing lower quality foods.

Daily Values: Ultimately, if a 2,000-calorie diet per day is not the amount of calories your body needs, than these numbers do not help you. Instead, use them as a general guide, but not the numbers you base your decision of purchasing. Also, when it comes to vitamins, simply stating "vitamin A" does not mean it is in the form your body needs or you would absorb all of the "110%" vitamin C, from orange juice, for example.

PACKAGING

Although we may know the right way to read a food label, ultimately the first thing we are faced with is the product packaging. Be careful not to fall for claims written on the front of the package. I ask patients to bring pictures of the packaging of products they are unsure of eating. In general, the first time they present me with a question about a product, they bring the front of the package. I explain to them the front does not help us decide if it is a quality food. "Yes, but it says *whole wheat*, or *fat free*, or *sugar free*," they may respond. I answer, "Those are the same reasons why I would put the product back on the shelf."

Here is why the claims on the front, for example, the claim that something is "All Natural," do not matter in our quest for packaged real food:

When a product claims to be fat free or sugar free or have zero grams of anything, it's most likely smart to stay away. The fundamental question is, "What are they putting in its place?" Usually, fat-free products have more sugar and chemicals to substitute for the fat flavor and stability. The sugar-free products probably have more fat and chemicals replacing the fundamentals of sugar in a product, like cohesion. A patient once called me while at the grocery store to ask which kind of pudding she should buy. Her choices were sugar free or fat free. I asked her to read the ingredients so we could see what was added in its place.

I asked her if there was another snack option she would like to eat or make it fresh, because these were not real-food choices. It is hard to make a better-quality decision when those are the options and you should not feel forced to make a poor choice. Try choosing another snack option that fits your health priorities instead of attempting to stick with products that do not fit your mold. Hopefully, your choice of *not* buying a product will influence others, and eventually the grocery store and food manufacturer will be forced to make a better-quality product. (We can only hope!)

Better-quality foods break down the different forms of nutrition facts on their packaging like fiber and fat specifics. The more you know about what you are eating, the better. Typically, when the company is sharing such detailed information by featuring a thorough break down of the nutrition facts label (this may include kinds of fiber and fats), it more likely means the company is not hiding anything in its products. When a product has healthful qualities, a company will take the opportunity to promote it. You shouldn't have to look too hard to see the healthy qualities on a food package; it will most likely be right in front of you. For example, when a product simply states "whole wheat" on the front of package, I would ask, "Why did they not say, *100 percent whole wheat*. If it was actually 100 percent whole wheat, they would say it."

Organic

Organic is similar to the concept of kosher since it is another word that developed flexibility in its definition and benefit for our health. Like kosher, not all organic foods are necessarily good for us. Just because a cookie is organic, does it mean it has less sugar, fewer carbs, less fat, or other ingredients than a non-organic cookie? No.

Oftentimes you see the news highlight studies on organic. (See the "Organic" section in chapter 7 for more information.)

I like to take every opportunity to lower the toxic load on my body. Our liver and kidneys create a natural detoxification system that filters out everyday toxins from our bodies that may be taken in by our environment, foods, and natural waste from bodily processes. Our bodies can only handle so much. If I can choose an organic food, like fruits and vegetables, and the price is right, I take advantage of it. I would never tell anyone to *not* eat fruits and vegetables because they are *not* organic. That is counterintuitive. In essence, when we eat a non-organic fruit or vegetable, we're getting more benefit from the anti-oxidant, anti-cancer properties and vitamins and minerals than if we were to not eat it. And we have no more permission to eat an organic cookie versus a non-organic one. But if I had a choice between organic and non-organic in a food I will buy regardless, I would choose one that is organic because it would decrease my toxic load and, typically, it would have better-quality, real-food ingredients.

INGREDIENTS

The reason why I am writing about ingredients after packaging is because ingredients will help us determine what to make of the claims on the front of the package. We can see a description of what is in our food and that is most important. The first three ingredients listed are in the highest amounts in the product. Ingredients like sugar should not be listed early on in the list, if at all. Another trick is when a product states that it is whole wheat on the front, but in the ingredients, it may read "enriched wheat flour, wheat flour, whole-wheat flour." It is mostly made from white flour and who really knows how much whole-wheat flour is included in the product. In his book *In Defense of Food: An Eater's Manifesto*, Michael Pollan suggests a great tactic while shopping is to try to choose foods with only five ingredients. I support making a more healthful choice by beginning to choose quality, packaged foods with the least amount of ingredients as possible on the label. Keep away from heavily processed preservatives like monosodium glutamate "MSG" and anything artificial, including flavors and colors.

The point is to try to find a food made with the most real-food ingredients as possible, in the smallest amount, minus all the chemicals, stabilizers, and preservatives. If you skim the ingredients and see a huge jumble of unpronounceable words that don't even look like real food, do yourself a huge health favor and put it back. Try and find a real-food option in the same category. Peanut and other nut butters are good examples of this. Nut

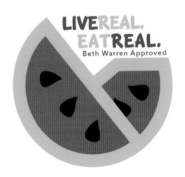

butters need only ingredients as close to "just nuts" as possible. You can more easily find this kind of nut butter amongst the other non-real-food options. Today, "natural" is listed on those varieties, but compare labels to find the best real-food option.

KOSHER CERTIFICATION

The kosher challenge is most intense when shopping for packaged foods. When picking up a product, you need to look for a kosher symbol (See chart on following page). There are many different kinds, designated by different rabbinical authorities. Consult your local rabbi for signs that are lawfully correct for your customs. If a product does not have a kosher certification or symbol, then it is not considered kosher by kashrut standards. Simply looking to see if it has kosher ingredients is not enough since it can be made amongst non-kosher ingredients and products and/or in a facility that makes non-kosher foods and risks cross-contamination.

Another valuable piece of information that comes along with a kosher symbol is a small letter D next to it. This factor easily distinguishes the product as being dairy. If you are avoiding dairy based on an allergy, this symbol is not always the most reliable dairy indicator. Sometimes a product was made in a facility with dairy and doesn't list dairy in the ingredients, so it is more important to read the ingredient list, as well. Formerly, there was a symbol DE (dairy equipment) next to the kosher symbol, which distinguished between actual dairy ingredients and the facility it was made in, but that abbreviation is no longer common. As a result of a D designation in a kosher diet, a dairy product should not be eaten with meat.

If D is not listed, or there is a P or Pareve listed next to the kosher symbol, then that means the product does not contain dairy ingredients. As a result, those keeping a kosher diet may eat the product with dairy foods.

KOSHER SYMBOLS

· · · · · · · · · · · · · · ·

A SAMPLING OF SOME KOSHER FOOD PACKAGING CERTIFICATIONS

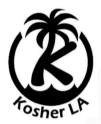

Kosher LA (Kola)

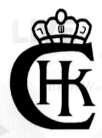

Beis Din of Crown Heights Vaad Hakashrus

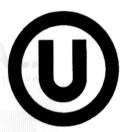

The Union of Orthodox Jewish Congregations (OU)

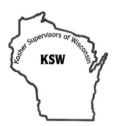

Kosher Supervisors of Wisconsin

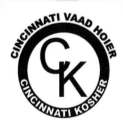

Cincinnati Vaad Hoier

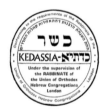

The Union of Orthodox Hebrew Congregations of London

These kosher symbols are for reference only. Consult your local rabbinical authority for your kashrut customs.

After you narrowed down your real-food choices with my other shopping tips, the deciding factor is kosher certification. Sometimes, this may mean none of your choices fit the bill, but you may be thankful for the push to make that product fresh or realize you had many other real-food options to purchase instead!

APPLYING WHAT YOU'VE LEARNED

LIVING A REAL LIFE: THE REAL FOOD KOSHER SHOPPING LIST

WE DID IT! I HOPE YOU ENJOYED YOUR REAL FOOD JOURNEY TOWARDS BETTER HEALTH! ONE OF MY MAJOR POINTS WAS TO FOCUS ON QUALITY OF CALORIES, NOT JUST QUANTITY. EATING A MAJORITY OF REAL FOOD IN YOUR DIET WILL HELP YOU MANAGE WEIGHT-LOSS AND HAS MANY OTHER HEALTH BENEFITS.

What to look for when buying packaged products:

1. Ingredients you can **pronounce.**
2. As **few** ingredients as possible.
3. **All natural** ingredients free of artificial colors and preservatives and harmful additives like MSG, hydrolyzed proteins, hydrogenated vegetable oils, and soy-based imitation foods.
4. **No added artificial sweeteners and limited natural,** real or artificial-Aspartame, NutraSweet, high fructose corn-syrup, agave nectar, refined white sugar, and cane sugar.
5. **To avoid GMOs** (Genetically Modified Organisms) corn, soy, sugar, zucchini, and papaya, should be certified organic. Limit cottonseed oil, corn oil, canola oil and grapeseed oil.
6. **Shop farmers' markets and food co-ops** for staples like nuts, olive oil, dairy products, and eggs in addition to fresh produce.
7. **Limit processed grain products** like breakfast cereals, granola, and store-bought baked goods that are highly processed. It is best to make your own. For example, oatmeal from steel-cut oats.

Real foods:

Examples of kosher brands are listed on the following pages, but others may meet the same criteria. **Consult your local rabbinical authority on validity of kosher symbols.**

Spices & Herbs

- ○ Allepo seasoning
- ○ Allspice
- ○ Basil
- ○ Bay Leaves
- ○ Black pepper
- ○ Cardamom
- ○ Caraway
- ○ Cayenne pepper
- ○ Chili pepper, dried
- ○ Cilantro/Coriander seeds
- ○ Cinnamon, ground
- ○ Cloves
- ○ Cumin seeds
- ○ Curry Powder
- ○ Dill
- ○ Garlic
- ○ Ginger
- ○ Italian seasoning
- ○ Mustard powder
- ○ Oregano
- ○ Parsley
- ○ Peppercorns
- ○ Peppermint
- ○ Poultry Seasoning
- ○ Rosemary
- ○ Saffron
- ○ Sage
- ○ Sea Salt—Celtic
- ○ Thyme
- ○ Turmeric
- ○ Anise Seeds OMint
- ○ Smoked Paprika
- ○ Hot Paprika
- ○ Nutmeg
- ○ Cloves
- ○ Zaatar

Vinegars

- ○ Raw apple cider vinegar (Braggs—KSA certified)
- ○ Raw coconut vinegar (Coconut Secret, Star-K)
- ○ Balsamic vinegar
- ○ Red Wine vinegar
- ○ Ume Plum Vinegar, Eden brand

Natural Sweeteners

- ○ Blackstrap molasses
- ○ Cane juice
- ○ Maple syrup
- ○ Brown rice syrup
- ○ Stevia
- ○ Xylitol (Natrazyle Honey Substitute)
- ○ Raw local honey
- ○ Coconut/palm sugar
- ○ Sucanat or Rapadura

Beverages

- ○ Green tea
- ○ Soy sauce, fermented
- ○ Tamari
- ○ Water
- ○ Sparkling water
- ○ Chamomile Tea
- ○ Rice milk
- ○ Kombucha (Synergy)
- ○ Kefir, coconut or diary

Grains / Cereals (3, Ideally 5+ grams fiber)/ Breads & Pasta (with 2+ grams fiber)

○ Amaranth
○ Barley
○ Brown rice
○ Buckwheat
○ Corn
○ Millet
○ Steel Cut Oats
○ Quinoa
○ Rye
○ Spelt Whole wheat
○ Cold cereals with over 5 grams of fiber
○ Granola
○ Muesli
○ Ezekiel brand
○ Barbara's brand, high fiber
○ Food for Life brand
○ Pasta from above grains or Tinkyada, Eden, Bionaturae 100% whole wheat
○ Organic Popcorn Organic Popcorn kernels
○ Basmati Rice
○ Jasmine Rice
○ Rice paper wrappers (Sushi Metsuyan)
○ Rice Pasta (Tinkyada) Buck-wheat Noodles
○ Quinoa
○ Whole grain crackers (Mary's Gone Crackers)

Beans, Legumes & Nuts

All beans—it is preferable to buy dried beans and soak overnight instead of buying canned beans.

○ Black beans Dried peas
○ Fava Beans
○ Garbanzo beans (chickpeas)
○ Kidney beans
○ Lentils
○ Lima beans
○ Miso
○ Navy beans
○ Pinto beans
○ Edamame
○ Tempeh
○ Tofu
○ Nuts & Seeds (raw) & Oils
○ Chia Seeds
○ Walnuts
○ Brazil nuts
○ Almonds
○ Cashews
○ Peanuts
○ Olive oil, extra virgin
○ Coconut oil, unrefined
○ Walnut oil Sesame oil
○ Avocado oil
○ Flaxseed Oil

- ○ Canola oil, organic
- ○ Macadamia nut oil
- ○ Pumpkin seeds
- ○ Flaxseeds, Milled (or grind "whole" in coffee grinder)
- ○ Sesame seeds
- ○ Sunflower seeds
- ○ Almond butter
- ○ Macadamia nut butter
- ○ Cashew butter
- ○ Walnut butter
- ○ Coconut butter/spread

Produce

Fruit

Fresh. Organic, if possible. Always keep lemons, limes, onions, garlic, ginger, parsley, cilantro, celery, and carrots around. They form the flavor foundation of so many dishes. Fresh is best, but frozen produce is also good. Avoid most store-bought canned fruits and vegetables.

- ○ **Apples**
- ○ Apricots
- ○ Bananas
- ○ Blueberries
- ○ Cantaloupe
- ○ **Cherries**
- ○ Cranberries
- ○ Figs
- ○ *Grapefruit*
- ○ **Grapes**
- ○ *Kiwifruit*
- ○ Lemon/Limes

- ○ *Mango*
- ○ **Nectarines**
- ○ Oranges
- ○ Papaya
- ○ **Peaches**
- ○ Pears
- ○ Pineapple
- ○ Plums
- ○ Prunes Raisins
- ○ Raspberries
- ○ **Strawberries**
- ○ Watermelon

Vegetables

- ○ *Asparagus*
- ○ *Avocados*
- ○ Beets
- ○ **Bell peppers**
- ○ Broccoli
- ○ Brussels sprouts
- ○ *Cabbage*
- ○ Carrots
- ○ Cauliflower
- ○ Celery
- ○ **Collard greens**
- ○ Corn
- ○ **Cucumbers**
- ○ *Eggplant*
- ○ Fennel

- ○ Garlic
- ○ Green beans
- ○ Green peas
- ○ **Hot peppers**
- ○ Kale
- ○ Leeks
- ○ *Mushrooms, crimini*
- ○ *Mushrooms, shiitake*
- ○ Mustard greens
- ○ Olives
- ○ *Onions*
- ○ **Potatoes**
- ○ Romaine lettuce
- ○ **Spinach**
- ○ **Squash, summer**
- ○ Squash, winter
- ○ *Sweet peas, frozen*
- ○ *Sweet potatoes*
- ○ Swiss chard
- ○ **Tomatoes**
- ○ Turnip greens
- ○ Yams

Dairy/Eggs
- ○ Cheese, low fat
- ○ Eggs—pastured best, organic, Omega-3 next best, free-range
- ○ Milk, cow's
- ○ Milk, goat's
- ○ Milk, coconut (not light) (Native Forest is BPA free)
- ○ Milk, almond
- ○ Yogurt, goat or cow, coconut, almond (Maple Hill Cream is grass-fed)
- ○ Kefir (Lifeway)

Poultry & Lean Meats
Grass-Fed or Pastured*, ideal
- ○ Beef
- ○ Lamb
- ○ Liver
- ○ Chicken
- ○ Turkey

Seafood (Wild, ideal)
- ○ Cod
- ○ Halibut
- ○ Salmon
- ○ Herring
- ○ Lemon of Sole
- ○ Flounder
- ○ Sustainably caught canned sardines, tuna, and salmon (Wild) Planet, Vital Cost-OU Certified and BPA-Free)
- ○ Wild-caught anchovies (Crown Prince—in glass jars and OU Certified)

Pantry
- ○ Marinara sauce—organic, no-sugar added, in glass jars (Middle Earth Organics, Seeds of Change)
- ○ Organic grape juice *(fruit*

juice should be limited- drink for the weekly Friday night/ Saturday lunch Shabbat or holiday blessings)

○ Red Wine, Kosher
○ Capers
○ Olives
○ Organic fruit spread—no added sugars (hard to find kosher, FiordiFrutta is kosher certified—sweetened with apple juice).

Make your own "quick jams" by cooking down fresh or frozen fruit, like blueberries until thick, season with citrus zest and raw honey if needed.

Baking Products
○ Blanched Almond Flour
○ Organic Sprouted Whole Grain Flour (To Your Health-Earth Kosher Certified)
○ Organic Sprouted Whole
○ Grain Brown Rice Flour (To Your Health)
○ Organic Unbleached White Flour
○ Coconut Flour
○ Tapioca FlourArrowroot
○ Instant yeast
○ Aluminum free baking soda
○ Aluminum free baking powder
○ Pure vanilla extract
○ Pure vanilla powder (Divine Organics)

○ Organic, 70% dark chocolate and chocolate chips (Ghirardelli, Sweetriot and Green & Black brands)
○ Organic cocoa powder
○ Unsweetened shredded coconut

Snacks
○ Raw nuts—almonds, pecans, walnuts, macadamia nuts.
○ Dried fruit (unsweetened and unsulphured)
○ Organic nut butters—almond, hazelnut (make homemade nutella with hazelnut butter, cocoa, raw honey or maple syrup)
○ Coconut flakes (Unsweetened)
○ Dried seaweed
○ Larabars
○ KIND Bars
○ PURE Bars
○ Think Thin Bars
○ Wild, brown rice cakes—eg. Lundenberg brand
○ Food Should Taste Good brand chips
○ Popcorn (Angies Delightfully Different) brand (Non-GMO)
○ Kale Chips (New York Naturals, Elvira's All Natural)

Refrigerator
○ Organic and Grass-fed meat and poultry, when possible
○ Pasture-raised eggs from farmers' markets or look for Vital Farms and Frenz's in the health food store.
○ Organic milk from grass-fed cows and not homogenized (Straus)
○ Organic milk plain yogurt (Maple Hill Cream)
○ Organic cream, preferably from grass-fed cows, and not ultra-pasteurized (Straus)
○ Organic butter from grass-fed cows (Strauss and Organic Valley Pasture Butter—OU Certified)
○ Clarified butter or ghee (Purity Farms is Kosher certified)
○ Grass-fed cheese
○ Bubbie's pickles
○ Homemade sauerkraut, or Bubbie's in markets (other brands are pasteurized).
○ Whole grain mustard, no added sugar
○ Organic salsa
○ Organic ketchup
○ Organic Yellow Mustard (Eden brand)
○ Hummus
○ Guacamole
○ Tallow - rendered beef fat (from grass-fed cows, available

from Kol Foods-NOT BEIT YOSEF to render at home) great for high heat cooking

Freezer
○ Organic fruit—no sugar added (great for smoothies)
○ Organic or *grass-fed meat
○ Organic or *pastured chicken
○ Chicken bones, feet, necks, etc (for homemade chicken stock)
○ Frozen sustainable fish fillets
○ Homemade frozen beef, chicken and fish stocks—or buy fresh fish stock from your local fish market and freeze for risottos and sushi rice (freeze in 2-cup pyrex containers or canning jars)
○ Frozen red/white wine (freeze leftover wine in jam jars)
○ Udi's whole grain products like buns, bread etc.
○ Brown rice or whole wheat 9-inch tortillas, like Ezekiel brand
○ Ground flaxseed
○ Coconut milk ice cream
○ Almond milk ice cream

○ Organic whole milk ice cream (the fewer ingredients the better), eg. Stonyfield

*Grow and Behold Kosher Pastured Meats and Kol Foods ship kosher certified (OU or Star-K BUT NOT BEIT YOSEF) pastured poultry and beef. They also have kosher nitrate-free sausages and hot dogs with only real ingredients. Look for a local buying club (or start your own).

Otherwise, stick to lean cuts of organic meat like London broil.

*SECONDARY SOURCE: REALFOODKOSHER.COM

MORE ON SNACKS

. . . .

Since snacking is a large part of living a real life with real food, here are ideas on how to make the perfect one. Remember, you should always combine a protein with a fiber. I call it "a fiber" because it can be either a 100% whole grain serving or a fruit. I recommend you choose fruit servings as the fiber portion of your snack most often and get in the habit of consuming it with a protein serving, which ensures your diet does not become too starchy. Some options, including edamame and nuts, technically have both fiber and protein. If you need to grab a quick snack, eat more of them (eg. 1 cup edamame or 1 oz of nuts, see below) instead of combining it with another protein or fiber option. Remember, snacks are "mini-meals." You can never go wrong with halving your protein and fiber servings from your meals to be used as a snack (like 2 oz of tuna and ¼ of a 100% whole wheat pita). All options below can be found in a brand with a kosher certification, and I referenced some of my favorites. The choices also abide by the kashrut principle of not mixing milk with meat foods.

SNACKING TIPS

. . . .

STEP ONE: FIGURE OUT WHAT YOU ARE CRAVING
What is it that you're craving, that's really going to satisfy you? Think about both the flavor and texture—are you craving salty or sweet, hot or chilled, creamy or crispy?

STEP TWO: THINK ABOUT MAKING A BETTER CHOICE, NOT A PERFECT CHOICE
Once you zero in on your craving, build the rest of your meal around your splurge. The goal is to make a better choice by identifying the food group of your splurge and pairing it with something better. To balance french fries, balance them out with veggies and a lean protein, like chicken or tofu. Similarly, baked goods or desserts can be

paired with fresh fruit. Pizza provides carbs, protein, and fat, but not enough veggies, so combining a slice with a salad dressed with balsamic vinegar would be a smart splurge strategy. Always ask yourself, how can I make this snack a better choice?

STEP THREE: SAVOR YOUR SPLURGE

Splurging can feel like cheating, which leads to an "on/off" mentality, but it is important to break that cycle. Building a smaller splurge into a relatively balanced meal makes much more sense than swinging back and forth between overeating and strictly dieting. A balanced approach allows for satisfaction without completely derailing your overall efforts. So slow down, enjoy every morsel, and finish your meal feeling content but not stuffed and sluggish. No matter what, finish the indulgence and get right back on track at your next meal or snack. The problem is not the one indulgence, but the negative effect it may have on your mind leading to more poor choices.

CHECK OUT THE MEAL PLANS FOR MORE SNACK OPTIONS

SNACKS (100-200 CALORIES)

•DAIRY   •MEAT   •PAREVE

- 4 oz. lowfat cottage cheese mixed with ¼ cup of diced fresh mango
- 1 small apple with 1 tablespoon natural peanut butter
- 15 baby carrots with 2 tablespoons of hummus
- One part-skim mozzarella cheese stick and a pear
- 6 oz. container of Greek yogurt: 140 calories
- 1 small banana with 8 raw walnuts
- Half a Larabar and 1 medium orange
- Trail mix made with 15 peanuts and a ¼ cup fiber-one or KIND granola
- Half a cup of shelled edamame drizzled with 2 tablespoons of Lemon Cumin Dressing

- ½ banana rolled in 1 tablespoon frozen >70% dark chocolate
- 1 package mango Matt's Munchies and 12 raw almonds
- 2 tablespoons almond butter with 4 stalks celery
- Yogurt parfait with 4 oz plain Greek yogurt, 2 tablespoons KIND granola and 1 cup mixed berries
- 1 KIND BAR (<200 calories for a snack)
- 1 oz raw nuts
- 2 tablespoons tehina with 3 carrots
- 5 olives and sliced cucumbers, 1 baby pack of whole wheat pretzels and 2 tablespoons hummus
- Ten Mary's Gone Crackers and ¼ avocado
- 1 cup unshelled edamame
- 18 baked whole grain tortilla chips with ¼ avocado
- 2 Lundenberg rice cakes, any variety, with ½ cup low-fat cottage cheese
- 1 oz dark chocolate (>70%) eg. Godiva, Green & Black
- 6 dark chocolate covered almonds (>70% dark chocolate)
- 1 latte with almond milk
- All-fruit ices made with 1 tablespoon almond butter
- 1–3 cups fresh popcorn with 1 tablespoon parmesan cheese
- Trail mix made with 15 peanuts and a mini box of raisins
- ½ cup of pumpkin seeds and 12 cherries
- 1 hard boiled egg
- 2 slices turkey ¼ whole wheat pita
- ½ cup cooked oatmeal with 4 walnut halves and ¼ cup blueberries
- Snack Smoothie: 1 cup fruit with 6 oz yogurt or milk
- "Food Should Taste Good" Multigrain Chips with ¼ cup fresh tomato salsa or Spicy Tomato Salad

MEAL PLANS

● ● ● ● ● ● ● ● ● ● ● ●

On the following pages are some sample meal plans that factor into living a real life with real food. Some key points to remember:

○ Always think about consuming a good quality protein and fiber in each meal and snack, with added non-starchy veggies, especially at lunch and dinner.

○ The plate model should be used as a guide for your lunch and dinner meals.

○ At dinnertime, the carbohydrate is optional, but if you typically have the nighttime munchies, make sure to include the whole grain carb at dinner.

○ The after-dinner snack is optional as well and is important to include if your typical night is grazing the cabinets in your kitchen and eating junky foods.

○ It is best to rotate your food choices for all meals and snacks, within the day, and alternated every three days.

○ The snack options can be swapped; the lunch and dinner options are interchangeable.

○ You may include coffee with breakfast without "counting it" as long as you use minimal milk (about 2 tbsp) and a natural sugar option, if needed (e.g. Agave or stevia 1 tsp).

○ Enjoy a 4-oz glass of red wine with dinner.

○ Get in the habit of drinking fennel or green tea after dinner and/or throughout the day.

○ Each food option follows the principles of the kosher diet, and you will not find a dairy dish within six hours of a meat option, or any dish with meat and milk mixed together.

○ There is no sequence to the weekly meal plans so you can choose which week you want to start with.

○ The "supercharge week" is a five-day meal plan that can be used when weight stabilizes for more than two weeks, or if you want to give your body a change to switch it up.

○ The meal plans represent five-days and you can choose to repeat one or two days as appropriate, leaving room for the Sabbath Friday night and Saturday lunch meals. (See Sabbath Meal Ideas for the Friday night and Saturday lunch meals, but keep all other meals and snacks as consistent as your week.)

○ The times indicated are suggested. It is better to get an early start on your day so you can fit in all the meals and snacks. If you wake up later, you may have to play around with the timing and the amount of food you are eating per day (e.g. omit a snack or start with lunch, etc).

○ Your body loves mealtime consistency, so try and make your sleep/wake cycle consistent.

• •

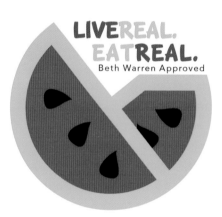

WEEK ONE

DAY 1	DAY 2	DAY 3	DAY 4	DAY 5
BREAKFAST 8:00 AM	**BREAKFAST 8:00 AM**	**BREAKFAST 8:00 AM**	**BREAKFAST 8:00 AM**	**BREAKFAST 8:00 AM**
¾ cup 1% cottage cheese with 1 c pineapple and 2 tsp flaxmeal	1 sl Sourdough French Toast with ½ cup berries	1 cup oatmeal, cooked with ½ cup blueberries and stevia (optional)	1 cup high-fiber cereal with 1 cup coconut milk and ½ grapefruit	Smoothie with 1 cup fruit, 1 tbsp almond butter, and 1 cup almond milk, unsweetened
SNACK 10:45 AM	**SNACK 10:45 AM**	**SNACK 10:45 AM**	**SNACK 10:45 AM**	**SNACK 10:45 AM**
1 PURE Bar <200 calories	3 celery sticks + 1 tbsp almond butter, natural	1 KIND Bar (170–180 calories)	1 sm orange + 9 cashews	2 pieces Eileen's Granola (¼ cup)
LUNCH 1:30 PM	**LUNCH 1:30 PM**	**LUNCH 1:30 PM**	**LUNCH 1:30 PM**	**LUNCH 1:30 PM**
Arugula Sesame Salad and 1 ½ cups Sherry's Lentil Soup	1½ cups Quinoa Salad with Israeli Salad	2 Easy Little Pizzas and Robyn's Fennel Salad	Spinach Salad with ½ cup Lentil Salad	2 Cheesy Spinach Portabellas and Allegra's Cabbage Salad
SNACK 3:45 PM	**SNACK 3:45 PM**	**SNACK 3:45 PM**	**SNACK 3:45 PM**	**SNACK 3:45 PM**
Green Smoothie with ½ cup kale, 1 cup spinach, 1 apple, and 8 walnuts	1 Hardboiled Egg +10 Mary's Gone Crackers	1 tbsp peanut butter, natural + 1 sm apple	2 Persian Cucumbers + 2tbsp Hummus with 1 tsp black/white sesame seeds	Trail Mix: ¼ cup high-fiber cereal, 10 peanuts, 2 tsp dark chocolate chips
DINNER 6:30 PM	**DINNER 6:30 PM**	**DINNER 6:30 PM**	**DINNER 6:30 PM**	**DINNER 6:30 PM**
½ cups Mujedre and 6 oz Greek Yogurt with Sarah's Kale Salad	4 oz Lemon Chicken with Hamid and ½ cup Beet Salad	2 Salmon Zaatar Skewers with ½ cup Syrian Potato Salad and side salad	Beef Goulash with a side of sautéed kale	½ cups Healthier Mac N Cheese with Dena's Soy Cabbage
AFTER DINNER (OPTIONAL) 8:30 PM	**AFTER DINNER (OPTIONAL) 8:30 PM**	**AFTER DINNER (OPTIONAL) 8:30 PM**	**AFTER DINNER (OPTIONAL) 8:30 PM**	**AFTER DINNER (OPTIONAL) 8:30 PM**
12 almonds, raw	1 c Dark Chocolate Popcorn	Fruit Salad: 1 cup fruit, 1 tsp lemon juice, 1 tsp coconut flakes, ½ tsp agave syrup, if needed	½ oz 70% dark chocolate	2 tbsp pumpkin seeds, unsalted ("Bizard")

WEEK TWO

DAY 1	DAY 2	DAY 3	DAY 4	DAY 5
BREAKFAST 8:00 AM	**BREAKFAST 8:00 AM**	**BREAKFAST 8:00 AM**	**BREAKFAST 8:00 AM**	**BREAKFAST 8:00 AM**
Kefir Smoothie: 2 ripe bananas, 1 cup vanilla kefir, and a pinch of cinnamon, nutmeg, allspice. Blend with ice.	Omelette with 2 whole eggs and 1 white, spinach, peppers, onions with 1 sl Ezekiel bread and ½ cup berries	2 Buckwheat Pancakes w/ ½ cup strawberries	2 tbsp almond butter on 2 brown rice cakes, topped with ½ banana	Lebne Mix: ¼ cup mango, 1 cup Lebne, 1 tsp chia seeds, a pinch of cinnamon or zaatar, ¼ tsp olive oil (optional) with ¼ whole wheat pita
SNACK 10:45 AM	**SNACK 10:45 AM**	**SNACK 10:45 AM**	**SNACK 10:45 AM**	**SNACK 10:45 AM**
1 KIND Bar (170-180 calories)	1 Chobani Pomegranate Greek Yogurt	1 brown rice cake + 1 tbsp almond butter, natural	1 part-skim cheese stick with 1 Mott's Munchies	12 almonds + 2 kiwis
LUNCH 1:30 PM	**LUNCH 1:30 PM**	**LUNCH 1:30 PM**	**LUNCH 1:30 PM**	**LUNCH 1:30 PM**
2 Veggie Burgers in ½ Damascus whole wheat pita bread with Cherise's Spicy Tomato Salad	1 Salmon Burger in Ezekiel Sesame Bun with Lettuce, Tomato, Onion, and Zucchini Sticks	Artichoke Gibbon and Fennel Soup	2 pieces Sarah's Pareve Yebra with Spinach Salad	4 oz Fish Sticks with Cherise's Spicy Tomato Salad
SNACK 3:45 PM	**SNACK 3:45 PM**	**SNACK 3:45 PM**	**SNACK 3:45 PM**	**SNACK 3:45 PM**
2 med carrots + 2 tbsp hummus	½ oz almond, raw + 1 apple	1 cup cantaloupe with ½ cup 1% cottage cheese	¼ avocado + 2 brown rice cakes	1 oz >70% dark chocolate
DINNER 6:30 PM	**DINNER 6:30 PM**	**DINNER 6:30 PM**	**DINNER 6:30 PM**	**DINNER 6:30 PM**
4 oz Pesto Crusted Salmon with sautéed spinach and ½ cup Wild Rice	1 piece Chicken with Okra with ½ cup Spanish Rice	½ cups Bulgur with Chickpeas with Dena's Soy Cabbage	4 oz Lemony Lemon of Sole with Garlicky String Beans	Stefanie's Chicken Soup with ½ cup Black Rice with Avocado Salad
AFTER DINNER (OPTIONAL) 8:30 PM	**AFTER DINNER (OPTIONAL) 8:30 PM**	**AFTER DINNER (OPTIONAL) 8:30 PM**	**AFTER DINNER (OPTIONAL) 8:30 PM**	**AFTER DINNER (OPTIONAL) 8:30 PM**
2 pieces Dark Chocolate Miniatures	1 oz sunflower seeds, unsalted	12 cherries	2 Clementines	5 Dark Chocolate Almonds

SUPERCHARGE WEEK

DAY 1	DAY 2	DAY 3	DAY 4	DAY 5
BREAKFAST 8:00 AM	**BREAKFAST 8:00 AM**	**BREAKFAST 8:00 AM**	**BREAKFAST 8:00 AM**	**BREAKFAST 8:00 AM**
1 cup lemon water (hot or cold) Squeeze juce from half lemon into water+ 1 cup oatmeal (1.5c cooked)+ ½ cup berries or 1 whole fruit w/1 tbsp flax meal	1 cup lemon water (hot or cold) Squeeze juce from half lemon into water+ 2 egg white + 1 yolk with diced veggies + 1 pear	1 cup lemon water (hot or cold) Squeeze juice from half lemon into water+ Smoothie: ¼ cup mango + ½ cup blackberries with 1 cup kale and stevia, if needed	1 cup lemon water (hot or cold) Squeeze juice from half lemon into water+Green Smoothie: 2 cups packed spinach, ½ cup kale, 1 apple, 16 walnut halves	1 cup lemon water (hot or cold) Squeeze juice from half lemon into water+1 cup oatmeal + ½ cup berries + 1 tbsp chia seeds
SNACK 10:45 AM	**SNACK 10:45AM**	**SNACK 10:45 AM**	**SNACK10:45AM**	**SNACK10:45AM**
½ cucumber + 2 tbsp hummus	23 raw almonds	1 celery stalk + 1 tbsp natural nut butter	8 baby carrots + 2 tbsp hummus	10 cherries +8 walnut halves
LUNCH 1:30 PM	**LUNCH 1:30 PM**	**LUNCH 1:30 PM**	**LUNCH 1:30 PM**	**LUNCH 1:30 PM**
1 cup green tea w/ 1 large salad (2tbsp dressing) +1½ cups Sherry's Lentil Soup	1 cup fennel tea with 1 large salad (2tbsp dressing) +1 cup Quinoa Salad	1 cup green tea with 1 large salad (2tbsp dressing) +1½ cups Chickpea Salad	My Veggie Burger with large salad (2 tbsp dressing) and 1 cup green tea	1 cup fennel tea + 1 salad + 1½ cups Beef Goulash
SNACK 3:45 PM	**SNACK 3:45 PM**	**SNACK 3:45 PM**	**SNACK 3:45 PM**	**SNACK 3:45 PM**
¼ cup dried fruit (no sugar or sulfite added) +8 walnuts	2 dates stuffed with almonds	2 cups Kale Chips + smoothie with 1 cup fruit and 1 cup almond milk	Trail Mix: ½ cup raw nuts + 2 tbsp sunflower or pumpkin seeds and ¼ dried fruit	2 square rice cakes + ¼ avocado
DINNER 6:30PM	**DINNER 6:30PM**	**DINNER 6:30PM**	**DINNER 6:30PM**	**DINNER 6:30PM**
4 oz chicken or turkey sandwich in Ezekiel corn tortilla, lettuce, tomato + 2 cups cruciferous veggies	5 ounces wild salmon, grilled + ½ cup brown rice and Dena's Soy Cabbage	2 Salmon Zaatar Skewers with 2 cups Allegra's Cabbage Salad	Cusa Gibbon + 3 cups asparagus, grilled, and ½ cup Beet Salad	4 oz grilled chicken + ½ sweet potato, baked + 3 cups string beans
AFTERDINNER (OPTIONAL) 8:30PM	**AFTERDINNER (OPTIONAL) 8:30PM**	**AFTERDINNER (OPTIONAL) 8:30PM**	**AFTERDINNER (OPTIONAL) 8:30PM**	**AFTERDINNER (OPTIONAL) 8:30PM**
1 orange	½ cup unsweetened apple sauce	2 tbsp sunflower seeds	1 small fruit cup, no added sugar	1 oz >70% dark chocolate

SABBATH MEAL OPTIONS:

A note about social meals, including the Sabbath:
As you learned in chapter 8, do not be overwhelmed by a meal with too many options. Keep in mind your plate model and fit the food choices into your plate. Want chicken and roast? No problem. Just be sure to fit both into one-quarter of your 9-inch plate. Rather have more chicken? Then leave out the roast. It's your choice. You are in charge—not the food. Oh yeah, and keep that challah to a minimum (2 oz for the blessing requirement), and make it whole wheat, unless you want it counting as the starch portion of your plate. Otherwise, you can always keep it simple with these real food options:

o Moroccan Fish with Vegetables and Brown Rice
o Chamin with salad
o Chulent with salad
o Chicken and Okra and Israeli Whole Grain Couscous
o Chicken and Potatoes with Garlicky String Beans
o Lemon Chicken with Spanish Rice and Arugula Salad
o Fasulia (Great Northern Beans with Marrow Bones and Meat) and Robyn's Fennel Salad
o Roast and Hamid with Wild Rice
o Hungarian Beef Goulash with 2 oz challah and salad

SABBATH DESSERTS:

Instead of throwing all your hard work toward better health down the drain on weekends (the all too familiar "We do not gain weight on the Sabbath" mantra), allow yourself one portioned indulgence as a part of your Sabbath routine, for one of your Sabbath meals (either Friday night or Saturday lunch, I recommend the latter because you are more active, awake and less likely to overindulge):
Healthy Apple Cobbler with 2 oz coconut ice cream, vanilla bean (optional)
6 dark chocolate covered almonds
4 pieces of fruit dipped in 1 oz dark chocolate
1 All Fruit Ices
1 cup Chocolate Popcorn

REAL-FOOD RECIPES

Here are some tasty real-food recipes that can easily fit into your real life and go along with my meal plans. With each recipe, a "plate tip" will guide you on how the dish fits into your meal so you can adapt a plan of your own. Most of the recipes take no longer than 20–30 minutes to prepare, some only 5–10 minutes! At times, you may have to adjust the servings to your taste, so feel free. For example, I love garlic, lemon, and cumin flavors, the base for most of these dishes, but you may want to scale up or down on the flavorings according to taste preference.

A lot of the recipes are from my Syrian roots, some from my Ashkenazic heritage, and others are simply ones I enjoy! A special thanks to many of my patients, friends, family, and go-to cooking sites for sharing some of their recipes, as well.

DRESSINGS, SAUCES, AND DIPS

These recipes for dips come from my Syrian roots. A great resource for these recipes and more of this style of cooking is *Aromas of Aleppo* by Poopa Dweck (also checkout Hamid and Fasulia recipes).

JULIA'S HUMMUS

Ingredients

¾ cup dried chickpeas (soaked in water overnight, refrigerated)
OR 2 - 15½ ounce cans of garbanzo beans
2–3 garlic cloves, peeled and chopped
3 tablespoons tahini paste

2 teaspoons cumin spice (adjust to taste)
½ teaspoon sea salt
Juice of 1–1½ lemons
3 tablespoons extra virgin olive oil
Water

Directions

Combine ingredients in food processor. Adjust flavorings to taste. Refrigerate for up to one week or freeze in ice cube trays for a quick, 2 tablespoon-sized snack.

Per serving (2 tablespoons): Calories 109; Fat 8.7 g (Saturated 1.2 g); Cholesterol 0 mg; Sodium 216.4 mg; Carbohydrate 9.3 g; Fiber 2.3 g; Protein 2.5 g

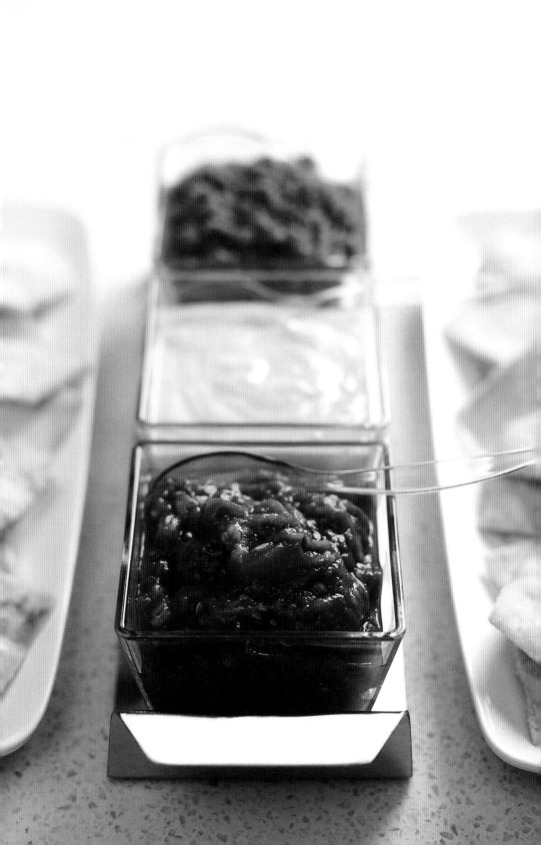

Spice Up Your Life: Garlic

Part of the allium family, and high in protective sulfur containing compounds, garlic is known to have many medicinal and other health benefits. In a 2007 study, garlic was shown to increase the synthesis of hydrogen sulfide inside our bodies, which acts as an antioxidant and transmits cellular signals that relax blood vessels and increase blood flow. The protective benefit may explain why a garlic-rich diet is shown to prevent breast, prostate, and colon cancers. Although it has been shown, inconsistently, to help lower cholesterol, researchers at the Albert Einstein School of Medicine injected garlic into mice, and found that it completely defended against heart muscle damage after a heart attack.

The protective benefits in a garlic-rich diet are ignited when consuming at least 2 medium-sized, whole garlic cloves per day. Lucky for us, recipes in Middle Eastern and Mediterranean cuisine (and many found in this book) call for garlic in most of the dishes.[118]

Although garlic may cause indigestion for some people, the most frequent complaint is about its influence on bad breath and sweat. Cooking with fennel seeds (see Fennel Salad) helps ward off some of the smell. Also, allow the garlic to sit for about 15 minutes after you crush the clove and before heating; this triggers an enzyme reaction that enhances the beneficial affects of the garlic.

EGGPLANT SALAD (MATBUCHA)

My sister, Adena, makes this recipe to go along with her Sabbath meals. I love the spicy flavor as an addition to any meal or added to sandwiches for more veggies. You may have to adjust the spicy flavoring to your taste.

Ingredients

1 large eggplant	1 jalapeño pepper
1 teaspoon salt	1 - 20 ounce can whole
4 cloves garlic	tomatoes
1 tablespoon extra	1 - 8 ounce can tomato sauce
virgin olive oil	Red pepper flakes, *optional*

Directions

Peel and dice eggplant. Place in strainer and sprinkle salt. Allow the juices to drip out. In a medium saucepan, sauté garlic, eggplant, jalapeño, and mash consistently. Add the can of tomatoes and tomato sauce, keep mashing. Add a sprinkle of red pepper flakes for more spice, if desired.

Per serving (2 tablespoons): Calories 61.3; Fat 2.6 g (Saturated 0.4 g); Cholesterol 0 mg; Sodium 591.7 mg; Carbohydrate 9.6 g; Fiber 2.9 g; Protein 1.7 g

TAHINA

● ●

Ingredients

3 cloves crushed garlic	½ cup tahini paste
2 tablespoons kosher salt	1 teaspoon cumin spice
Juice of 2-3 lemons	

Directions

Purée garlic in a food processor, then add in remaining ingredients. Adjust flavorings to taste. Refrigerate up to one week or freeze in ice cube trays for quick, 2-tablespoon snacks.

Per serving (2 tablespoons): Calories 92; Fat 8.2 g (Saturated 1.1 g); Cholesterol 0 mg; Sodium 588.3 mg; Carbohydrate 8.5 g; Fiber 2.6 g; Protein 3.1 g

BAZARGAN

● ● ● ● ● ● ● ● ● ● ● ● ● ● ● ● ● ● ● ●

Ingredients

1 cup fine bulgur (cracked wheat) soaked in hot water for about 15 minutes (drain excess water)

1 small onion, chopped

Juice of 1 lemon

2 tablespoons tomato paste

8 tablespoons Out

OR tamarind concentrate, available in specialty stores or some supermarkets

5 tablespoons extra virgin olive oil

2 teaspoons cumin spice

Kosher salt

½ cup chopped walnuts for garnish

Directions

Place bulgur in mixing bowl and add all the ingredients. Stir to combine. Adjust seasoning to taste.

Per serving (2 tablespoons): Calories 151; Fat 11.2 g (Saturated 1.4 g); Cholesterol 0 mg; Sodium 85.8 mg; Carbohydrate 12.9 g; Fiber 1.6 g; Protein 2.2 g

---

Spice Up Your Life: Onions

Onions are part of the alliaceous family—along with garlic, leeks, shallots, and chives. The high sulfur content reduces carcinogenic effects of nitrosamines and N-nitroso compounds found in over-grilled meat. They also promote apoptosis (cell death) in colon, breast, lung, and prostate cancer and in cases of leukemia. We can see that onions were a part of the Israelite diet when they were slaves in Egypt because they reminisced of those days eating onions in Egypt in the Book of Numbers (11:5). Onions are rich in phytonutrients, like quercetin, and minerals, like chromium, which are linked to improving mood and insulin function and promoting blood sugar control.

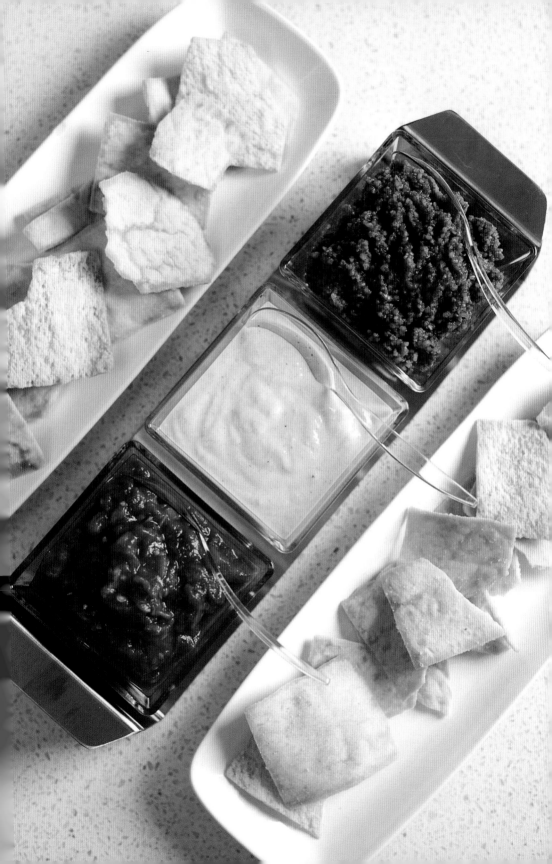

VEGETABLES

Each dish can be used towards your non-starchy vegetable portion on your plate (½ the plate), unless otherwise noted. In each salad, you may add 2 tablespoons of your choice of dressing from my real-food recipes.

LACTO-FERMENTED VEGETABLES ("PICKLING")

• •

As discussed in chapter 7, the art of lacto-fermentation falls more in line with the traditional pickling of Eastern European Jewry and is less like those of Spanish descent who may use vinegar in their pickling methods. Here is how Tom Malterre, author of *The Whole Life Nutrition Cookbook* and creator of nourishinghope.com, pickles his vegetables to extract the most probiotic benefits:

Ingredients

1 glass quart jar with a plastic lid   2 cups filtered water
1–1½ tablespoon sea salt

Any Combination of Raw Organic Vegetables:

chopped cauliflower   chopped carrots   chopped bell peppers
chopped beets   chopped green beans   sliced radishes

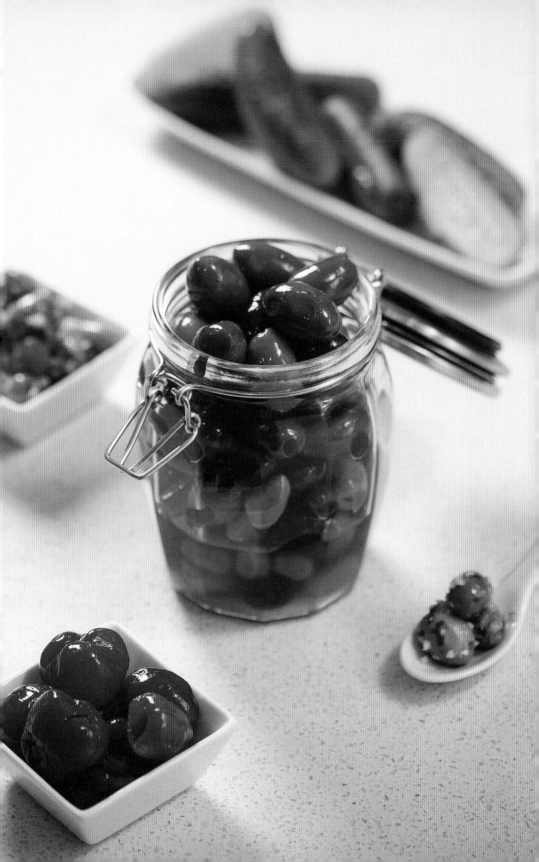

sliced daikon	chopped kale	cabbage leaves (for the
sliced cucumbers	chopped onions	top)
chopped turnips	chopped green onions	
chopped broccoli	chopped garlic	

Any Combination of Herbs and Spices:

dried chili peppers	fresh basil	sea vegetables (arame
black peppercorns	fresh tarragon	or hijiki)—use less salt
bay leaf	fresh mint	if using these
fresh dill		

Directions

Dissolve your sea salt in water in a glass jar or 2-cup glass measure.

Place your favorite combination of vegetables into a quart jar. (You can use a larger cylindrical jar or ceramic crock instead, just double or triple the salt brine keeping the same ratio of salt and water.) Add a few layers of herbs and spices, too. (Tom prefers the peppercorns in the first layer, on the bottom of the jar, so they don't float to the top.) Make sure you leave about an inch from the top of the jar.

Cover with your salt brine, leaving about 1-inch to a ½-inch from the top. Fold a small cabbage leaf and press it into the brine so the water floats above it and the vegetables are completely submerged. Cover with a plastic lid (it's best not to use metal, as the salt and acids can corrode it, though you may occasionally use it if it's all you have). Don't screw the lid on too tight; you want some space for gasses to release. You should see a bit of bubbling and some liquid possibly dripping out after the third day, depending on the heat level in your home.

You may place jars into some sort of container, like a rectangular casserole dish, to catch any drips. Set your jars in an undisturbed place in your kitchen—out of direct sunlight—for example, on top of the refrigerator.

You can taste the veggies after about five days to see how soured they are. A good rule of thumb is to allow the vegetables to ferment for about seven to eight days in the winter and five to six days in late summer—sometimes in the summer, they can sit for even ten or more days. Just experiment; there is no exact science with fermentation. After your veggies are soured to your liking, remove the cabbage leaf and place the jar (or jars) in your refrigerator where they will store for months.

Use your vegetables on top of cooked quinoa, beans, and chopped leafy greens. Serve them atop grilled fish or chicken. Serve them with scrambled eggs for breakfast. And try to restrain yourself from eating the whole jar in one sitting—it may be a little too much salt all at once! You can also whisk some of the leftover brine with olive oil, a squirt of Dijon mustard, and a dash of honey for a probiotic salad dressing!
Source: www.NourishingMeals.com

ARUGULA SESAME SALAD

Serves 4

Ingredients

Arugula (1-5 ounce container of
   Organic Girl Arugula)

1 tablespoon sesame seeds

1 tablespoon sunflower seeds

1 tablespoon pumpkin
   seeds

¼ cup cranberries

¼ cup walnuts, chopped

Directions

Toast sesame seeds, pumpkin seeds, and sunflower seeds for 3–5 minutes. Combine all ingredients in salad bowl (careful not to burn!). Add 2 tablespoons of Balsamic Dressing.

Per serving: **Calories 90; Fat 7.5 g (Saturated 0.8 g); Cholesterol 0 mg; Sodium 15.7 mg; Carbohydrate 4.6 g; Fiber 2.0 g; Protein 3.2 g**

SARAH'S KALE SALAD

● ●

Serves 4

Ingredients

Salad

1 bunch kale, chopped

1 small red onion, sliced

½ red pepper, thinly sliced

1 tablespoon mixed black and
    white sesame seeds

Dressing

2 teaspoons Ume plum vinegar
    (e.g., Eden Foods® brand)

1 teaspoon extra virgin
    olive oil

2 tablespoons water

Directions

Combine all ingredients in salad bowl. Mix in dressing.

Per serving: Calories 57; Fat 1.6 g (Saturated 0.3 g); Cholesterol 0 mg; Sodium 291.8 mg; Carbohydrate 8.0 g; Fiber 1.8 g; Protein 2.7 g

---

A note on Ume Plum Vinegar

Eden Foods® makes the Ume Plum Vinegar, which is a by-product of fermenting umeboshi plums originating from Japan. Because of the high salt needed to achieve the right acid balance for fermentation, be sure not to add salt to your meal with this dish and be mindful of the portion (see chapter 7).

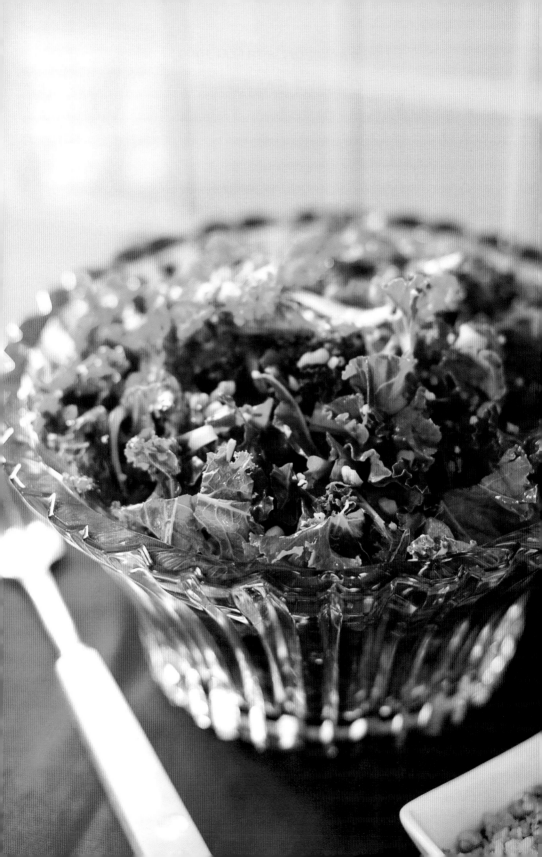

BEET SALAD

• •

Serves 4

Ingredients

6 beets

1 tablespoon extra virgin
olive oil

3 tablespoon lemon juice,
freshly squeezed

1 tablespoon cumin

1 teaspoon Kosher salt

½ cup flat leaf parsley, finely
chopped

½ small onion, chopped

Directions

Place beets in saucepan, cover with water and boil. Reduce heat to low
and simmer for 15 minutes or until the beets are fork tender. Drain the
beets and rinse under cold water to stop the cooking process. Rub off the
skin of the beets with a paper towel. Cut the beets in cubes and transfer
to mixing bowl. In a separate bowl, combine olive oil, lemon, cumin, and
salt. Mix in onions and parsley. Add dressing and adjust to taste.

Per serving: Calories 97.4; Fat 4.1 g (Saturated 0.6 g); Cholesterol 0 mg; Sodium
686.6 mg; Carbohydrate 14.5 g; Fiber 4.1 g; Protein 2.6 g

CHICKPEA SALAD

• •

Serves 4

Ingredients

¾ cup fresh chickpeas (soak them
overnight about 6–8 hours,
then boil until fork-tender.
Peel off outer shells.)
OR 1–15-ounce can of chickpeas,
rinsed

1 scallion, chopped

1 stalk celery, chopped

2 tablespoons flat leaf parsley,
chopped

2 tablespoons extra virgin
olive oil

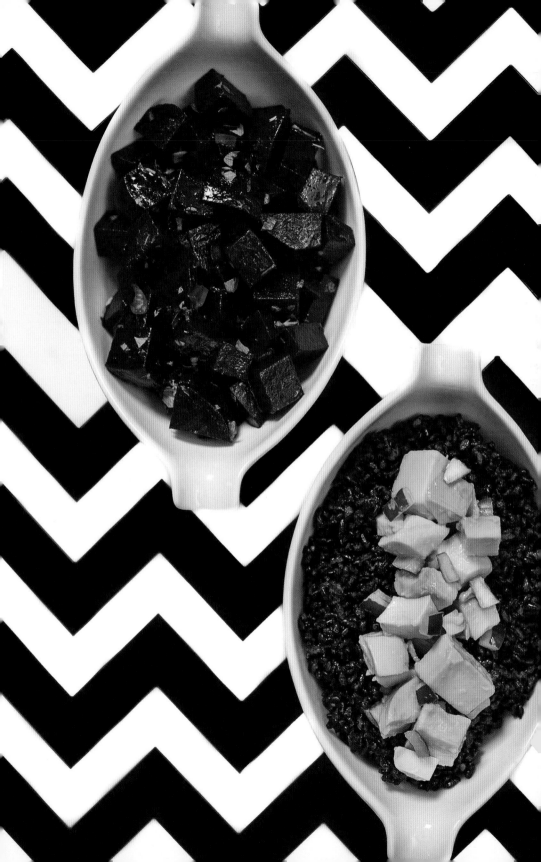

1 teaspoon cumin

¼ teaspoon salt

Dash of white pepper

Juice of 1 lemon

Directions

Combine ingredients in medium glass mixing bowl. Stir well. Adjust seasonings to taste.

Per serving: Calories 123.2; Fat 7.7 g (Saturated 1.1 g); Cholesterol 0 mg; Sodium 292.6 mg; Carbohydrate 12.4 g; Fiber 2.6 g; Protein 2.6 g

---

Spice Up Your Life: Parsley

Parsley is an excellent source of vitamin A, vitamin C, and vitamin K. It is a good source of iron and folate. Because of the oils and flavonoids, not only do parsley properties act as antioxidants, but they increase the antioxidant capacity inside the cell.[119]

SYRIAN POTATO SALAD

• •

Serves 6

Ingredients

6 medium potatoes*

1 teaspoon ground cumin

¼ cup extra virgin olive oil

1 teaspoon kosher salt

¾ cup freshly squeezed lemon
  juice

2 hard boiled eggs,
  sliced

1 teaspoon ground allspice

4 scallions, chopped

*I leave the peels on for added fiber and nutrients, along with lowering the glycemic index of the potatoes.

Directions

Boil the potatoes in large pot until tender, about 20 minutes. Cut the potatoes in small squares and place in medium mixing bowl. Add the

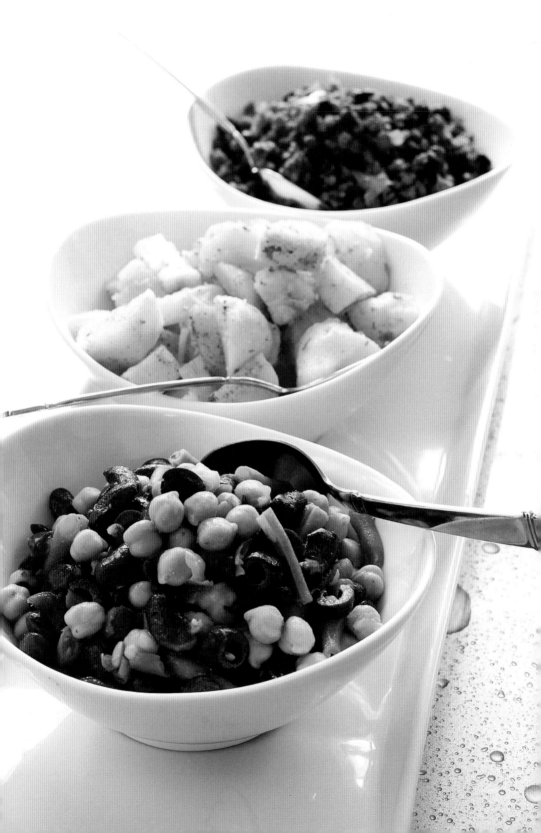

olive oil and lemon juice, then the seasonings. Gently mix the potatoes and place sliced eggs on top.

Per serving: Calories 226; Fat 11.3 g (Saturated 1.9 g); Cholesterol 62.0 mg; Sodium 415.4 mg; Carbohydrate 26.8 g; Fiber 3.2 g; Protein 6.2 g

---

Spice Up Your Life: Scallions and Allspice

Scallions are part of the allium family (which includes garlic, onions, chives, and leeks) and have anti-cancer and anti-inflammatory benefits.[120]

Allspice acts as an anti-inflammatory, rubefacient (warming and soothing), carminative, and anti-flatulent spice. It has health-benefiting essential oils, which gives pleasant, sweet aromatic fragrances to this spice. It also contains caryophyllene, methyleugenol, glycosides, tannins, quercetin, resin, and sesquiterpenes. Similar to black peppercorns, the active principles in the allspice may increase the motility of the gastro-intestinal tract as well as enhancing digestion by increasing enzyme secretions inside the stomach and intestines. Eugenol has local anesthetic and antiseptic properties.

Studies have shown that preparations made from allspice oil mixed with extractions from garlic, and oregano can work against E.coli, Salmonella, and L.monocytogenes infections.

Allspice contains vitamin A, vitamin B-6 (pyridoxine), riboflavin, niacin and vitamin-C and the minerals potassium, manganese, iron, copper, selenium, and magnesium.

ISRAELI SALAD

* *

Serves 4

Ingredients

3 tomatoes, diced

4 Persian cucumbers, diced

1 red pepper, diced

1 yellow pepper, diced

1 green pepper, diced

1 bunch flat leaf parsley, chopped

Juice of 1 lemon

¼ teaspoon salt

2 cloves garlic, crushed

Dash of black pepper

1 tablespoon extra virgin
   olive oil

Directions

Combine all ingredients in medium glass mixing bowl. Dress the salad with seasonings and adjust to taste.

Per serving: Calories 117.4; Fat 4.5 g (Saturated 0.5 g); Cholesterol 0 mg; Sodium 154.1 mg; Carbohydrate 26.0 g; Fiber 2.9 g; Protein 3.1 g

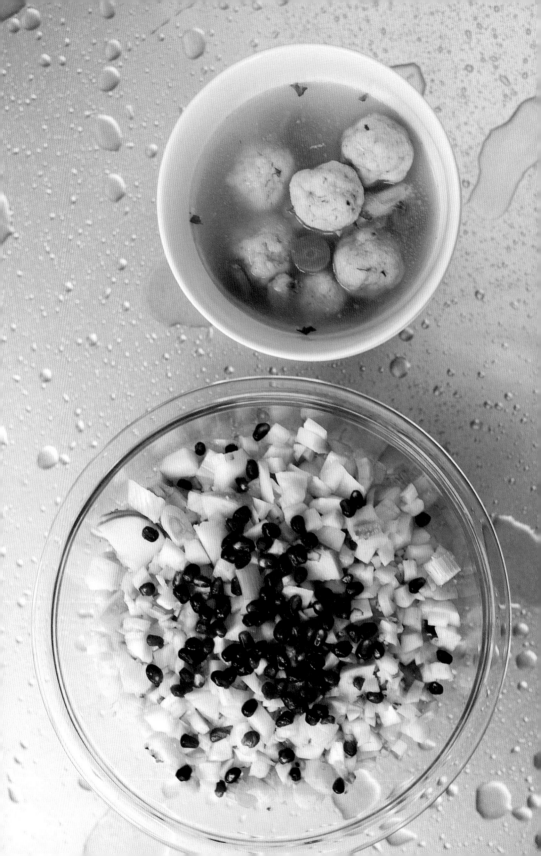

ROBYN'S FENNEL SALAD

● ● ● ● ● ● ● ● ● ● ● ● ● ● ● ● ● ● ● ●

Serves 4

Ingredients

2 bulbs fennel, chopped

½ thinly sliced green apple

¼ cup pomegranate seeds

Juice of ½ lime

1 tablespoon chopped walnuts

Salt and pepper, to taste

Directions

Combine ingredients in glass mixing bowl. Sprinkle salt and pepper to taste.

Per serving: Calories 67.4; Fat 1.5 g (Saturated 0.1 g); Cholesterol 0 mg; Sodium 100.1 mg; Carbohydrate 13.7 g; Fiber 4.3 g; Protein 1.9 g

SPINACH SALAD

● ● ● ● ● ● ● ● ● ● ● ● ● ● ● ● ● ● ● ●

Serves 4

Ingredients

2 bags baby spinach

3 hard boiled eggs, sliced

¼ red onion, sliced

Lemon Cumin Dressing

Directions

Combine ingredients in glass mixing bowl.

Per serving: Calories 94.2; Fat 4.5 g (Saturated 1.3 g); Cholesterol 139.5 mg; Sodium 158.9 mg; Carbohydrate 6.3 g; Fiber 3.2 g; Protein 8.9 g

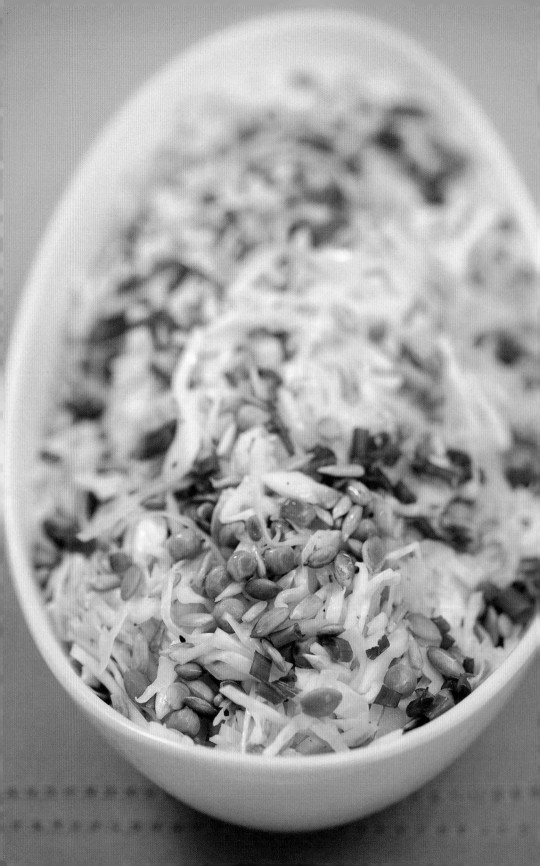

ALLEGRA'S CABBAGE SALAD

Serves 4

Ingredients

1 head cabbage, shredded
finely

1 bag frozen peas

¼ cup pumpkin seeds

¼ cup sunflower seeds

Scallions or chives, chopped,
optional

Juice of 1½ lemons

1 tablespoon extra virgin olive oil

Salt and pepper to taste

Directions

Combine ingredients in glass mixing bowl. Stir in lemon juice and oil. Sprinkle salt and pepper to taste.

Per serving: Calories 231; Fat 9.4 g (Saturated 1.2 g); Cholesterol 0 mg; Sodium 197.9 mg; Carbohydrate 32.3 g; Fiber 11.7 g; Protein 10.5 g

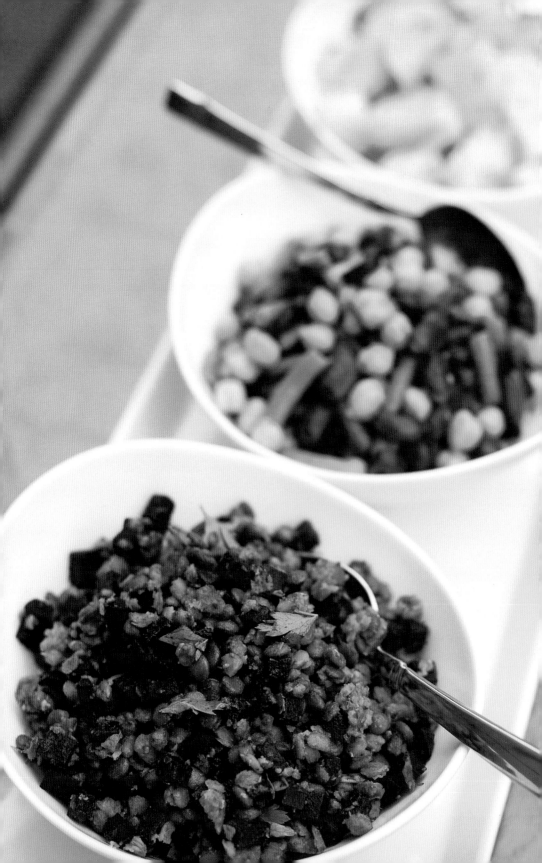

BEAN SALAD

• •

Serves 12

Ingredients

1 15-ounce can kidney beans

1 15 ½-ounce can chickpeas

1 15-ounce can black beans

1 cup steamed string beans, chopped

2 tablespoons red wine vinegar

1 tablespoon extra virgin olive oil

Salt, pepper, and garlic powder, to taste

Directions

Combine all legumes (rinse and drain). Combine vinegar, oil, salt, pepper, and garlic powder and stir. Pour over beans. Adjust to taste.

Per serving (½ cup): Calories 133.6; Fat 1.9g (Saturated 0.3g); Cholesterol 0 mg; Sodium 296.9 g; Carbohydrate 23.1 g; Fiber 7.3 g; Protein 6.9 g

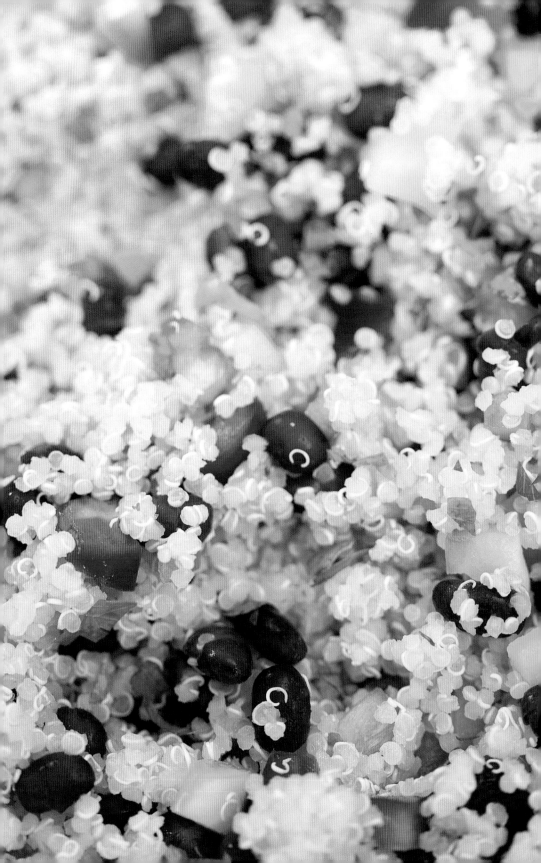

QUINOA SALAD

• •

Serves 6

Ingredients

1 cup quinoa, uncooked
(red or white)

1 red bell pepper, chopped

1 green bell pepper, chopped

1 orange bell pepper,
chopped

1 15-ounce can black beans

1 2.25-ounce can sliced black
olives

1 tablespoon cilantro, chopped

Lemon juice, to taste

¼ teaspoon salt

Dash of Pepper

1 tablespoon extra virgin olive oil

Directions

Cook quinoa according to package directions. Combine all ingredients.
Adjust to taste.

Per serving: **Calories 229.5; Fat 5.7 g (Saturated 0.4 g); Cholesterol 0 mg; Sodium
29.4 mg; Carbohydrate 39.2 g; Fiber 9.2 g; Protein 11.0 g**

Spice Up Your Life: Cilantro

The leaf component of parsley was found to have a higher concentration of phenolic compounds than cilantro. One study showed
that the phenolic compounds extracted from both parsley and
cilantro are responsible, in part, for both antioxidant and antibac-
terial activities.[121]

CHEESY SPINACH PORTABELLAS

Serves 4

Ingredients

1 cup fresh spinach, finely
  chopped

½ cup part-skim mozzarella cheese

½ teaspoon garlic powder

¾ cup prepared marinara sauce

4 large Portobello mushroom caps

¼ teaspoon salt

¼ teaspoon freshly ground pepper,
  divided

1 cup part-skim ricotta cheese

Directions

Preheat oven to 450° F. Coat a rimmed baking sheet with cooking spray. Place mushroom caps, gill-side up, on the prepared pan. Sprinkle with salt and ⅛ teaspoon pepper. Roast until tender, 20—25 minutes.

Mash ricotta, spinach, ¼ cup mozzarella, garlic powder, and the remaining ⅛ teaspoon pepper in a medium bowl.

When the mushrooms are tender, carefully pour out any liquid accumulated in the caps. Return the caps to the pan gill-side up. Spread 1 tablespoon marinara into each cap; cover the remaining sauce to keep warm. Mound a generous ⅓ cup ricotta filling into each cap and sprinkle with the remaining ¼ cup Parmesan.

Bake until hot, about 10 minutes. Serve with the remaining marinara sauce.

Adapted from: Eatingwell.com.

Per serving: **Calories 212.8; Fat 10.6 g (Saturated 6.0 g); Sodium 553.5 mg; Carbohydrate 13.5 g; Fiber 2.5 g; Protein 17.3 g**

KUSA JIBBON (SQUASH AND CHEESE)

Serves 12

Ingredients

2 pounds zucchini or yellow
   squash, chopped

1 small onion, finely chopped

1 teaspoon extra virgin olive oil

3 egg whites and 1 whole egg,
   beaten

6 ounces part-skim muenster
   cheese

½ cup low-fat cottage cheese

1 teaspoon sea salt

Directions

Preheat oven to 350° F. Sauté the squash and onion with olive oil in a large skillet for about 8 minutes. In a separate mixing bowl, combine the eggs, cheese, cottage cheese, and salt with the squash and onion mixture. Stir to combine. Pour into 2-quart baking dish, or 12 individual soufflé cups.

Per serving: Calories 97.6; Fat 5.7 g (Saturated 0.4 g); Cholesterol 34.5 mg; Sodium 307.0 mg; Carbohydrate 4.4 g; Fiber 1.2 g; Protein 6.9 g

Adapted from: Aromas of Allepo.

LENTIL SALAD

● ●

Serves 4

Ingredients

2 cups lentils (any color)

4 cups water

3 fresh beets

Juice of 1 lemon

¼ teaspoon salt

1 teaspoon cumin

1 tablespoon extra virgin
    olive oil

1 tablespoon cilantro, fresh

½ teaspoon salt

Directions

Add water and lentils into a medium saucepan. Bring the water to a rapid simmer over medium-high heat, then reduce the heat. Cook, uncovered, for 20-30 minutes. Add water as needed to make sure the lentils are just barely covered. Separately, boil beets, peel and chop in cubes. Combine lentils with beets in mixing bowl. Add salt, cumin, oil, cilantro, and salt. Stir to combine. Stir just before serving. Adjust seasonings to taste.

Per serving: Calories 174.2; Fat 4.0 g (Saturated 0.6 g); Cholesterol 0 mg; Sodium 490.8 mg; Carbohydrate 26.9 g; Fiber 9.6 g; Protein 10.1 g

GARLICKY STRING BEANS

* *

Serves 2

Ingredients

1 tablespoon sesame oil

1 pound string beans

1 tablespoon white sesame seeds

4 cloves garlic, minced

Salt, to taste

Directions

Heat oil in skillet. Add garlic and sauté until translucent. Add string beans and continuously stir-fry until crisp-tender. Turn off heat, sprinkle salt, and mix in sesame seeds.

Per serving: Calories 139.9; Fat 9.0 g (Saturated 1.3 g); Cholesterol 0 mg; Sodium 2.5 mg; Carbohydrate 10.6 g; Fiber 3.7 g; Protein 1.2 g

ZUCCHINI STICKS

● ●

Serves 8

Ingredients

3 large zucchini (about 1½ pounds)

½ cup dry whole-wheat matzo meal

⅓ cup flaxmeal

½ cup whole grain panko (e.g., Ian's® Japanese whole grain breadcrumbs)

¼ cup (1 oz.) grated fresh parmesan cheese

½ teaspoon salt

⅛ teaspoon freshly ground black pepper

½ cup egg substitute or 1 egg, beaten

4 tablespoons water

Directions

Preheat oven to 400° F.

To prepare zucchini: cut zucchini, 1 at a time, in half crosswise; cut each half lengthwise into 8 wedges.

Combine breadcrumbs, panko, cheese, ½ teaspoon salt, and black pepper in a shallow dish. Dip zucchini in egg with 4 tablespoons water, dredge in breadcrumb mixture. Place zucchini on a wire rack coated with cooking spray. Lightly coat zucchini with cooking spray.

Bake at 400° F for 25 minutes or until golden brown. Serve immediately with sauce.

Per serving: Calories 67.7; Fat 1.6 g (Saturated 0.9 g); Cholesterol 23.3 mg; Sodium 81.6 mg; Carbohydrate 6.4 g; Fiber 1.5 g; Protein 3.4 g

DENA'S SOY CABBAGE

● ●

Serves 4

Ingredients

1 head cabbage, chopped

3 teaspoons extra virgin
  olive oil

1 tablespoon water

⅛ cup soy sauce

Salt, to taste

Directions

Place cabbage in a roaster. Drizzle on oil, water, soy sauce, and salt. Stir to combine. Cover tightly and bake at 350° F for about 1–1 ½ hours.

Per serving: Calories 48.4; Fat 3.6 g (Saturated 0.5 g); Cholesterol 0 mg; Sodium 498.2 mg; Carbohydrate 3.9 g; Fiber 1.4 g; Protein 1.3 g

CHERISE'S SPICY TOMATO SALAD

● ●

Serves 2

Ingredients

1 10 ½ – ounce container cherry
  tomatoes, sliced in halves

1 long hot pepper, seeded and
  chopped

Juice of 1 lemon

¼ teaspoon salt

Dash of white pepper

1 tablespoon extra virgin
  olive oil

2 cloves garlic, minced

Directions

Combine ingredients in medium glass mixing bowl. Adjust seasoning to taste.

Per serving: Calories 80; Fat 7.0 g (Saturated 1.0 g); Cholesterol 0 mg; Sodium 290.9 mg; Carbohydrate 5.5 g; Fiber 0.1 g; Protein 0.1 g

STARCHES

SARAH'S PAREVE YEBRA (STUFFED GRAPELEAVES)

● ● ● ● ● ● ● ● ● ● ● ● ● ● ● ● ● ● ● ●

Serves 6

Ingredients

Filling

2–3 shallots, chopped

1 teaspoon plus 1 tablespoon
   extra virgin olive oil,
   separated

1 cup quinoa

2 cups water

1 bunch fresh parsley, chopped

Salt and pepper to taste

Dash cinnamon

3–4 tablespoons *Ou**

1 bunch dried prunes
   (a small handful)

1 bunch dried apricots
   (a small handful)

Sauce

1 cup lemon juice

½ cup extra virgin olive oil

8 cloves of garlic, crushed

2 tablespoons of salt

2 tablespoons agave syrup

1 handful of mint

**Ou* is available at some groceries
   and specialty supermarkets,
   and may be referred to as,
   Tamarhindi.

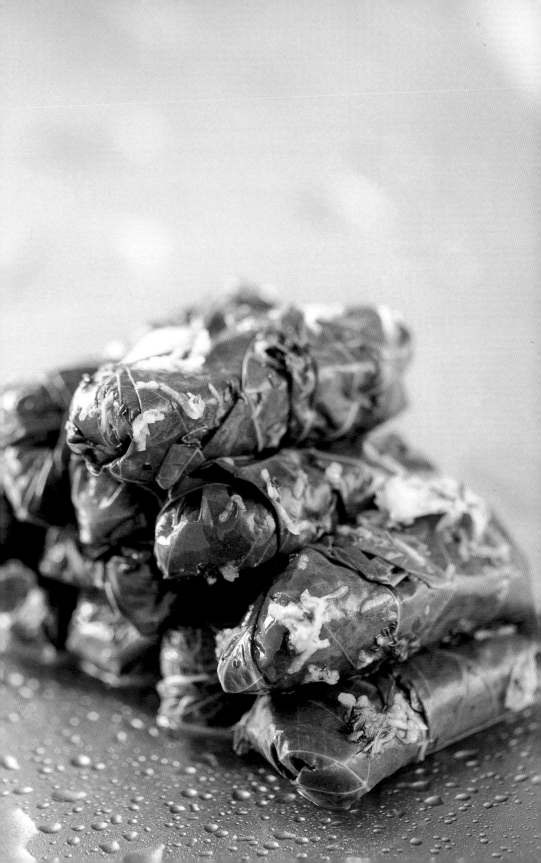

Directions

Filling:

Sautee 2–3 shallots in extra virgin olive oil. Separately, cook 1 cup quinoa in 2 cups water, boil and simmer until water evaporates. Combine parsley and ou into quinoa and add salt, pepper and cinnamon. Place apricots and prunes in food processor until paste-like consistency. Mix into quinoa with shallots.

Grape Leaves:

Cut off tips of leaves. Scoop 1 tablespoon of filling a few inches below the leaves and roll into cigar-like shapes.

Blend the sauce ingredients together in food processor. Layer stuffed grape leaves in a glass 7-¼"L x 6-⅝"W square casserole dish. Pour in the sauce. Cover the dish and bake at 350° F for 1 hour.

Per serving (Stuffed Grapeleave): Calories 193.9; Fat 3.4 g (Saturated 0.4 g); Cholesterol 0 mg; Sodium 30.2 mg; Carbohydrate 37.4 g; Fiber 3.3 g; Protein 5.1 g

Per serving (Sauce): Calories 181.5; Fat 18.7 (Saturated 2.7 g); Cholesterol 0 mg; Sodium 2,327.2 mg; Carbohydrate 4.8 g; Fiber 0.3 g; Fiber 0.3 g; Protein 0.4 g

MUJEDRE (RICE AND LENTILS)

Serves 8

Ingredients

1 cup lentils

2 cups brown rice

1 medium onion

1 tablespoon extra virgin
olive oil

Salt and pepper to taste

Directions

Sauté chopped onion in oil. Set aside. Put 1 cup of water on high heat and lentils. Cover the pot for the lentils to soften and there is no more water left. Cook the rice per package directions, in about 4 cups of water, and add in lentils, onion, salt, and pepper. Stir to combine.

Serving Suggestion: Serve with 6 ounces plain Greek yogurt and sautéed spinach.

Per serving: Calories 93.5; Fat 1.1 g (Saturated 0.2 g); Cholesterol 0 mg; Sodium 1.4 mg; Carbohydrate 17.6 g; Fiber 3.1 g; Protein 3.5 g

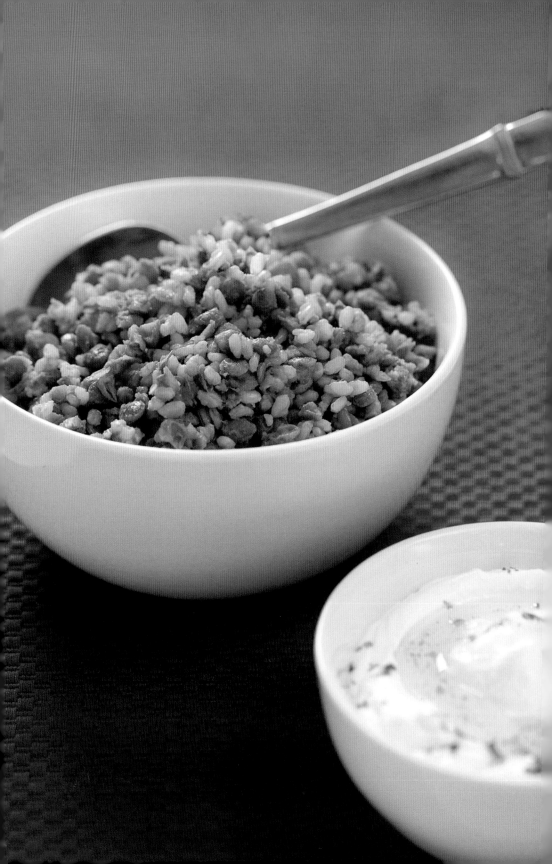

SPANISH RICE

● ●

Serves 6

Ingredients

1 cup brown rice or whole
   grain orzo

2 cups water

16 ounces marinara sauce

1 - 16-ounce bag frozen mixed
   vegetables

1 medium onion,
   minced

1 tablespoon extra virgin
   olive oil

Salt and pepper, to taste

Directions

Sauté onion in oil over medium heat. When onion becomes translucent and starts to brown, add rice, water, marinara, vegetables, salt, and pepper. Stir and cover. Reduce heat to low flame and cook until there is no more water. Transfer to 9¼ x 5¼-inch rectangle casserole dish, and place in oven on 350° F for 10 minutes if you like it to be crispy.

Per serving: Calories 170.7; Fat 5.7 g (Saturated 0.8 g); Cholesterol 0.0 mg; Sodium 580.5 mg; Carbohydrate 26.7 g; Fiber 5.0 g; Protein 4.5 g

WILD RICE

● ● ● ● ● ● ● ● ● ● ● ● ● ● ● ● ● ● ●

Serves 6

Ingredients

¼ cup sliced almonds

1 cup wild rice

¼ cup fresh cranberry sauce

OR ¼ cup dried cranberries
(sulfite free, no
added sugar)

Directions

Make 1 cup of wild rice according to package directions. After you add the rice and water, mix in ¼ cup almond slices, cook until al dente. Stir in ¼ cup of fresh cranberry sauce or dried cranberries.

> To make cranberry sauce, you'll need ¼ cup xylitol, 3 cups fresh cranberries (one package), and ¼ cup water. Boil together, about 4 minutes. Set in glass bowl, cover with saran wrap, and chill in the refrigerator.

Per serving (including sauce): Calories 77.8; Fat 2.7 g (Saturated 0.2 g); Cholesterol 0.0 mg; Sodium 1.8 mg; Carbohydrate 12.6 g; Fiber 3.2 g; Protein 2.4 g

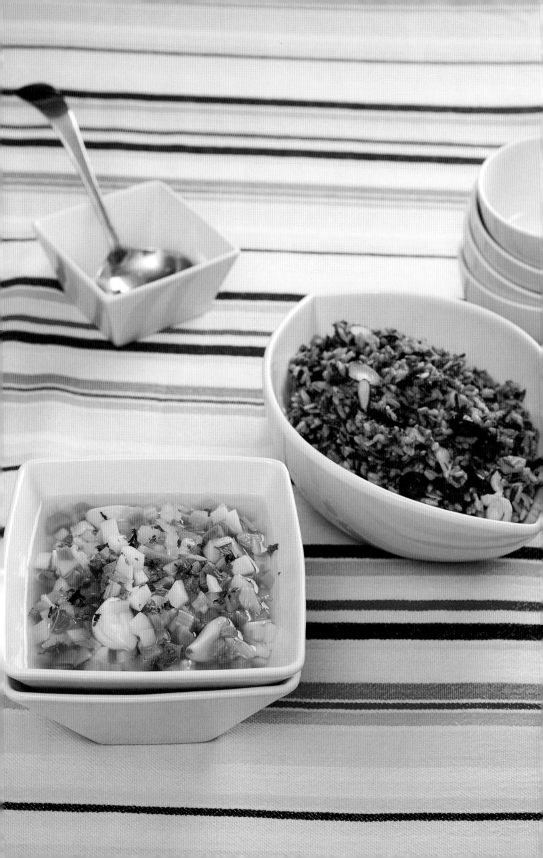

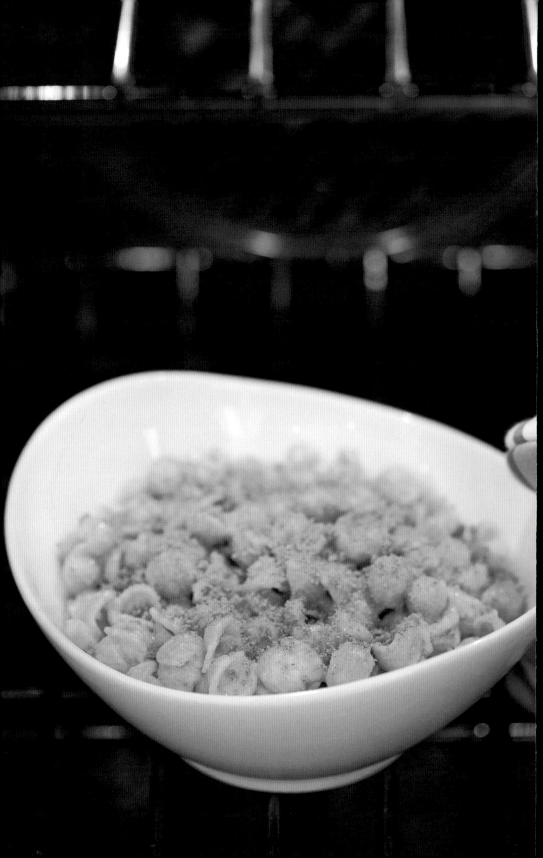

HEALTHIER MAC 'N' CHEESE

* * * * * * * * * * * * * * * * * * * *

Serves 9

Ingredients

1½ cups whole-wheat elbow
   noodle

Nonstick cooking spray

1 tablespoon whole-wheat flour

1 teaspoon coconut oil

½ cup skim milk

¾ cup part-skim mozzarella
   cheese

¾ cup part-skim muenster cheese

½ teaspoon salt

½ teaspoon garlic powder

⅛ teaspoon black pepper

2 tablespoon whole-wheat panko
   crumbs

1 12-ounce bag of frozen
   cauliflower

Directions

Steam cauliflower; purée and drain in cheese-cloth or colander. Heat coconut oil in pot. Stir in flour, continuously, to make a roux. Add in the milk and allow to thicken (approximately 4 minutes). Add all spices. Whisk in the cheese, a little at time, in a figure-8 motion. Turn off the heat.

Stir in cauliflower purée, add pasta back in and whisk in the cheese sauce. Put noodles in 9-¼"L x 5-¼"W rectangle casserole dish, sprinkle with whole-wheat panko crumbs, and bake at 350° F for 15 minutes.

Per serving: Calories 138; Fat 7.1 g; (Saturated Fat 4.5 g); Cholesterol 22.1 mg; Sodium 307.5 mg; Carbohydrate 9.9 g; Fiber 2.1 g; Protein 9.9 g

BLACK RICE

There's not much to this one—just cook according to package directions! Try serving black rice with Avocado Salad to mix things up.

AVOCADO SALAD

Serves 2

Ingredients

1 Avocado

Juice of 1 lemon

½ teaspoon garlic powder

1 teaspoon cumin

½ teaspoon salt

Red onion, chopped, optional for garnish

Directions

Peel and cut avocado into large chunks. Season with lemon juice, garlic powder, cumin, and salt. Garnish with red onion, if desired.

Per serving: Calories 190; Fat 14.8; (Saturated Fat 2.2 g); Cholesterol 0.0 mg; Sodium 582.8 mg; Carbohydrate 14.1 g; Fiber 7.5 g; Protein 2.6 g

EASY LITTLE PIZZAS

● ● ● ● ● ● ● ● ● ● ● ● ● ● ● ● ● ● ● ●

Serves 12

Ingredients

1 package of whole-wheat mini pizza dough (24 pack)

Marinara sauce (about ½ 24-ounce jar)

18 ounce package of part-skim mozzarella cheese

Oregano, garlic powder, and red pepper flakes, to taste

Directions

Place parchment paper on two baking sheets and put each frozen dough on the parchment paper, separated. Put 1 teaspoon of sauce on each dough, followed by 1 tablespoon of cheese, and spread over the dough. Add oregano, garlic powder and red pepper flakes to taste. Bake for 10–12 minutes on 350˚ F.

For a different flavor, omit the sauce and add zaatar spice on top of the cheese for zaatar pizzas.

Want an even healthier real food version? Omit the cheese and add your choice of vegetables and olives in its place! The omission of cheese makes the recipe pareve.

Per serving: **Calories 148.8; Fat 4.8g (Saturated 2.2 g); Cholesterol 11 mg; Sodium 259.7 mg; Carbohydrate 18.3 g; Fiber 1.2 g; Protein 7.7 g**

BULGUR WITH CHICKPEAS

● ● ● ● ● ● ● ● ● ● ● ● ● ● ● ● ● ● ● ●

Serves 6

Ingredients

½ cup cracked bulgur

1 cup boiling water

Coarse salt and freshly ground
   pepper

1 - 15-ounce can chickpeas, rinsed
   and drained

1 scallion, thinly sliced

½ cup fresh mint leaves, torn if large

2 medium carrots, peeled and
   chopped (1 cup)

¼ teaspoon chopped garlic
   (about 1 small clove)

¼ cup shelled pistachios,
   toasted

¼ cup extra virgin olive oil

1 lemon wedge

Directions

In saucepan, cook one part bulgur to two parts water; bring water to a boil, add bulgur, stir for 2 minutes. Remove from heat, cover; let stand for 4 minutes; drain excess water. Fluff with a fork. Stir in chickpeas, scallion, and mint.

Separately, pulse carrots, garlic, and pistachios in a food processor until coarsely chopped, forming a pesto sauce. Drizzle in oil and process until combined. Season with salt and pepper. Stir pesto sauce into bulgur mixture, squeeze with lemon and adjust to taste.

Per serving: Calories 190.4; Fat 10.2 g (Saturated 1.4 g); Cholesterol 0.1 mg; Sodium 229.8 mg; Carbohydrates 21.9 g; Fiber 5.1 g; Protein 4.3 g

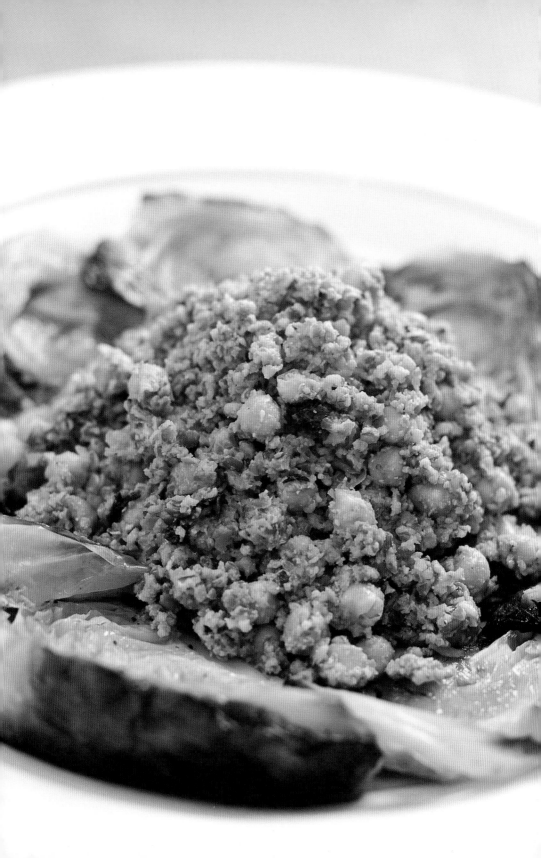

Spice Up Your Life: Mint

Mint is linked to aiding indigestion because it calms the muscles of the stomach and improves the flow of bile, which the body uses to digest fats. Therefore, it helps with weight loss because it allows the food to pass through your stomach more quickly.

One study examined fifty-seven people with IBS who received either enteric-coated peppermint capsules or placebo twice a day for four weeks. Of the people who took peppermint, 75 percent had a significant reduction of IBS symptoms[122] (the actual mint leaves and oil can cause indigestion for IBS and GERD conditions). Peppermint may help improve tension headaches by calming the muscles in the forehead and temples, too!

Peppermint and its main active agent, menthol, are great decongestants. Because menthol thins mucus, it is also a good expectorant, which means it helps loosen phlegm and breaks up coughs. It is soothing and calming for sore throats (pharyngitis) and dry coughs, as well.[123]

PROTEINS

LEMON CHICKEN

* *

Serves 4

Ingredients

1 pound chicken cutlets

1 cup whole-wheat matzo meal

1 teaspoon paprika

1 teaspoon salt

½ teaspoon pepper

Juice of 1 lemon and rind
    separately

14 ounces of organic chicken stock

Directions

Combine matzo meal with salt, pepper, and paprika in a bowl. Squirt half of lemon juice onto the chicken cutlets, and dip the chicken cutlets, one at a time, into the matzo meal mixture.

    In a heated cast-iron skillet, put 1 tablespoon canola oil. Add chicken and brown lightly on both sides. Put chicken into rectangle casserole dish and grate lemon rind on top. Add organic chicken stock on top and bake for 30 minutes on 350° F to cook the inside of the chicken.

Per serving: Calories 228.8; Fat 3.0 g (Saturated 0.8 g); Cholesterol 62.4 mg; Sodium 648.7 mg; Carbohydrate 29.5 g; Fiber 1.3 g; Protein 18.9 g

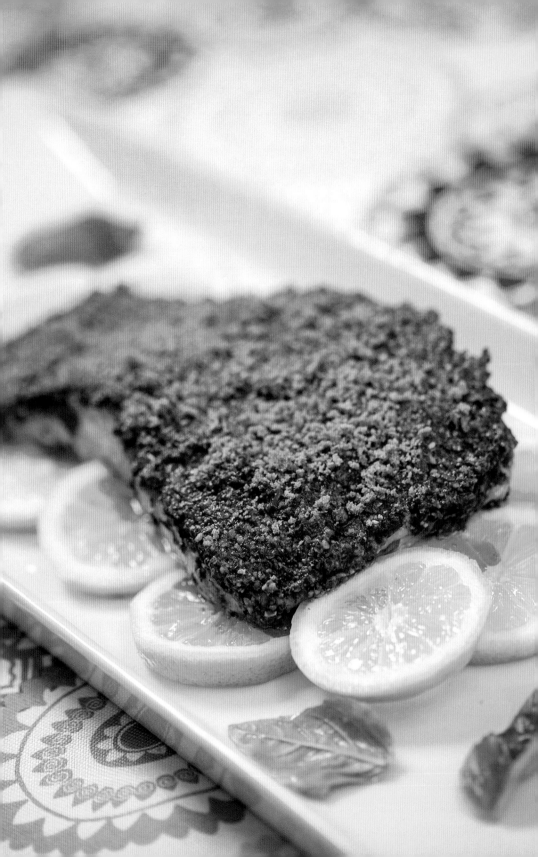

PESTO CRUSTED SALMON

• •

Serves 4

Ingredients

1 pound wild salmon,
   with the skin
½ fresh lemon

2 tablespoons of Walnut Pesto Sauce
4 tablespoons whole-wheat panko
   crumbs (optional)

Directions

Line baking tray with parchment paper, lay the fish, skin side down. Squeeze half lemon over the fish, spread on pesto sauce to cover top and sides of the fish. Sprinkle panko crumbs on top. Broil for 5 minutes and then bake for about 15 minutes on 350° F or until inside is flaky, not sticky.

Per serving: Calories 209.3; Fat 9.9 g (Saturated 1.7 g); Cholesterol 64.8 mg; Sodium 111.1 mg; Carbohydrates 4.6 g; Fiber 0.8 g; Protein 24.0 g

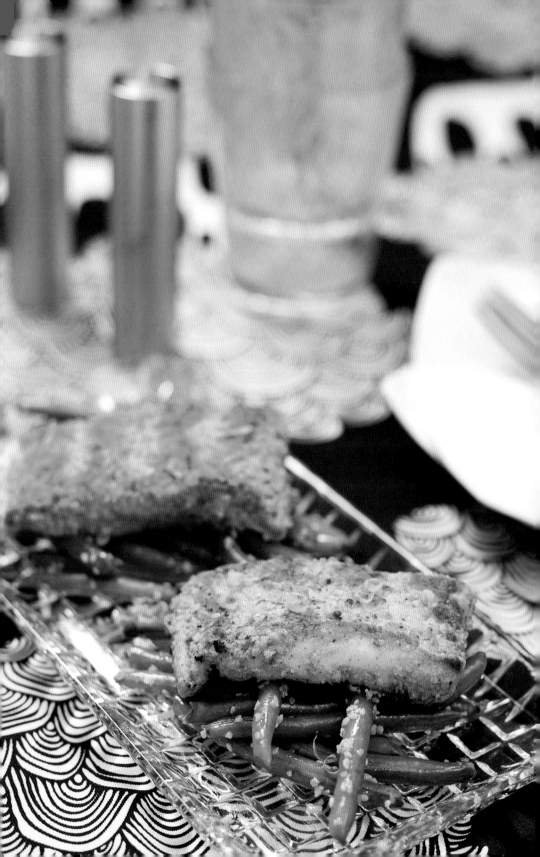

LEMONY, LEMON OF SOLE

• •

Serves 4

Ingredients

1 pound lemon of sole

⅓ cup whole-wheat flour

1 teaspoon flaxmeal

1 lemon, juice and rind

Salt and pepper, to taste

1 tablespoon organic canola oil

Directions

Combine flour, flaxmeal, salt, and pepper on plate. In a separate bowl, squeeze ½ lemon on the pieces of fish, dip each side in the flour mixture. Heat oil in skillet. Place fish into the skillet, and cook about one minute on each side. Put on baking sheet lined with parchment paper and squeeze the other half of lemon over the fish. Grate lemon rind from both halves over the fish. Bake on 350° F for about 7 minutes until the inside of the fish is flaky.

Per serving: Calories 374; Fat 15.3 g (Saturated 2.2 g); Cholesterol 64.8 mg; Sodium 111.1 mg; Carbohydrate 12.9 g; Fiber 2.1 g; Protein 45.1 g

VEGGIE BURGER

Serves 8

Ingredients

2 teaspoons chia seeds

3 tablespoons warm water

1 medium onion

6 ounces mushroom

3 cloves garlic

2 cups cooked lentils, drained

⅓ cup old-fashioned oats

1 tablespoon tamari

1 tablespoon tomato paste

Oregano, basil, smoked paprika, salt, thyme, and pepper, to taste

Directions

Put chia in warm water, set the bowl aside. Mince mushrooms and garlic in food processor, sauté onion in skillet. Stir in mushrooms and garlic and add 1 tablespoon water. Cover until mushrooms soften. Transfer to food processor, add lentils and chia seeds. Pulse to combine.

Set for 15 minutes then mold into small patties and put on baking sheet. Bake on 375° F for 30 minutes.

Per serving: **Calories 104.5; Fat 0.9g (Saturated 0.1 g); Cholesterol 0.0 mg; Sodium 298.8 mg; Carbohydrate 18.9 g; Fiber 6.1 g; Protein 7.1 g**

Adapted from: fatfreevegan.com.

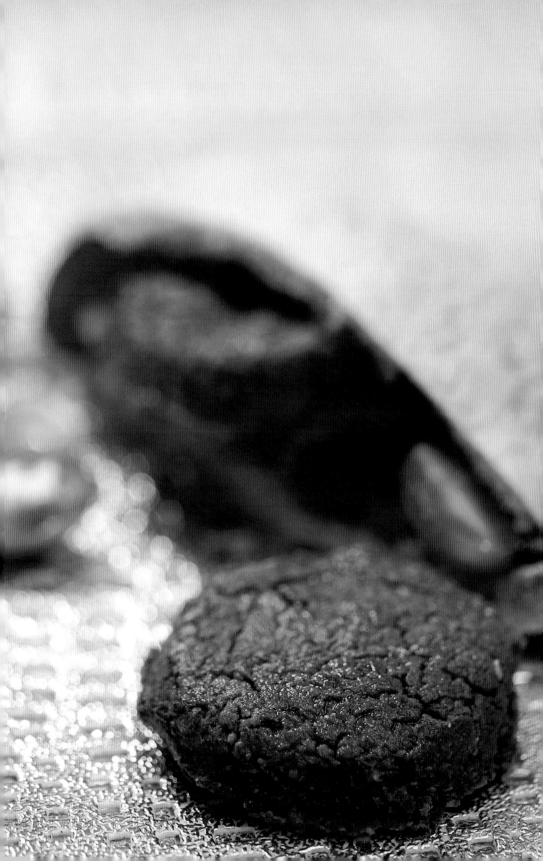

SALMON ZA'ATAR SKEWERS

Serves 8

Ingredients

2 pounds wild salmon*, skinless, cubed

3 limes

¼ cup za'atar spice

⅓ cup extra virgin olive oil

4 green bell peppers, cubed

4 red bell peppers, cubed

3 onions, cubed

Grape tomatoes

Wooden skewers

*I chose the fish with its own "meat" and the most absorbed form of Omega-3 healthy fat, EPA and DHA (see chapter 4).

Directions

In small bowl, combine zaatar spice, juice of 3 limes, and oil as dressing and stir to combine. Take 1 skewer and slide on an onion, red pepper, green pepper, and salmon cube, and repeat three times. Top with a grape tomato.

Place completed skewers in small baking dish. Brush dressing on salmon skewers. Pour in remaining dressing, cover with plastic wrap and refrigerate for at least 4 hours. Place on heated grill (or broil in oven) and cook 5–10 minutes on each side

Per serving: Calories 324.2; Fat 17.0 g (Saturated 2.5 g); Cholesterol 62.7 mg; Sodium 79.2 mg; Carbohydrate 19.0 mg; Fiber 5.0 g; Protein 25.0 g

For a complete and nutritionally balanced meal, serve with grilled asparagus (pg TK) and wild rice (pg TK) or healthy mac n cheese (pg TK).

Spice Up Your Life: Za'atar

Tying in my Sephardic Jewry to the dish, the zaatar spice is frequently used in Mediterranean dishes. Za'atar is generally prepared using ground dried thyme, oregano, marjoram, or some combination thereof, mixed with toasted sesame seeds and salt, though other spices such as sumac might also be added. It can easily be bought already prepared from Middle Eastern specialty stores and some supermarkets.

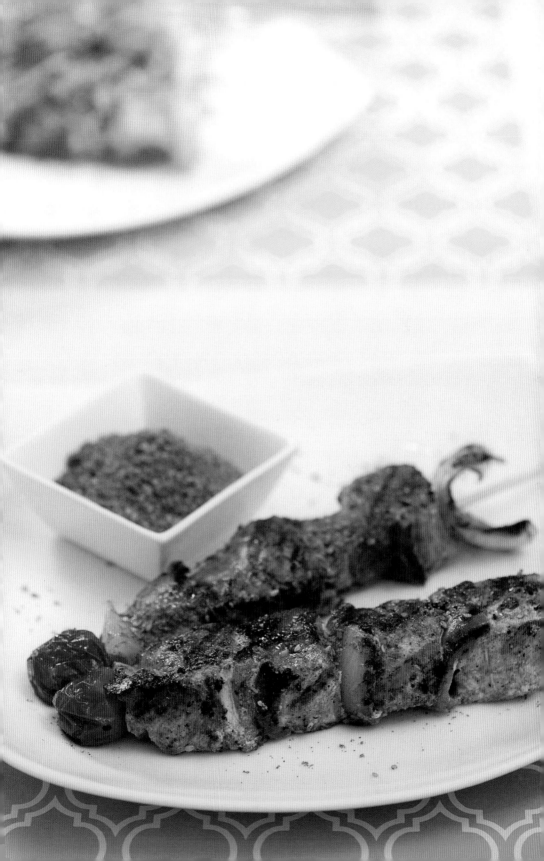

BEEF GOULASH

• •

This beef goulash is a hit every time. I tweaked the recipe from *Better Homes and Garden* magazine and it is a perfect, balanced dish for meat lovers.

Serves 8

Ingredients

2 pounds grass-fed beef stew meat (such as chuck), trimmed and cubed

2 teaspoon caraway seeds

1½–2 tablespoon sweet or hot paprika (or a mixture of the two)

¼ teaspoon salt

Freshly ground pepper, to taste

1 large onion, chopped

1 small red bell pepper, chopped

1 - 14-ounce can diced tomatoes

1 - 14-ounce can reduced-sodium beef broth

1 teaspoon Worcestershire sauce

3 cloves garlic, minced

2 bay leaves

2 tablespoons fresh parsley, chopped

Directions

Place beef in a 4-quart or larger slow cooker. Crush caraway seeds with the bottom of a saucepan. Transfer to a small bowl and stir in paprika, salt, and pepper. Sprinkle the beef with the spice mixture and toss to coat well. Top with onion and bell pepper.

Combine tomatoes, broth, Worcestershire sauce, and garlic in a medium saucepan; bring to a simmer. Pour over the beef and vegetables. Place bay leaves on top. Cover and cook until the beef is very tender, 4–4½ hours on high, or 7–7½ hours on low.

Discard the bay leaves; skim or blot any visible fat from the surface of the stew. Serve sprinkled with parsley.

Tips

Make Ahead Tip: Cover and refrigerate for up to two days or freeze for up to four months.

Prep ahead: Trim beef and coat with spice mixture. Prepare vegetables. Combine tomatoes, broth, Worcestershire sauce, and garlic. Refrigerate in separate covered containers for up to one day.

Per serving (one cup): 180 calories; 5 g fat (2 g sat , 2 g mono); 48 mg cholesterol; 6 g carbohydrates; 0 g added sugars; 25 g protein; 1 g fiber; 250 mg sodium; 298 mg potassium. Nutrition Bonus: Zinc (40 percent daily value), Vitamin C (35% dv), Vitamin A (25% dv), Iron (15% dv).

Spice Up Your Life: Peppermint and Caraway

A combination of essential oils (peppermint and caraway) have an amazing ability to soothe gastrointestinal upset. Both were shown to allow smooth muscle relaxation of the stomach and duodenum. In a double-blind, placebo-controlled trial with forty-five patients, researchers found improved symptoms of indigestion, including sensations of pressure, heaviness, and fullness, in 89.5 percent of the population.[124]

SALMON BURGER

● ●

A great alternative to the hamburger, this burger is a great way to try a salmon dish.

Serves 8

Ingredients

2 pounds wild salmon, ground

2 tablespoons fresh cilantro, chopped

1 scallion, chopped

Juice from ½ of a lemon

1 teaspoon garlic powder

1 teaspoon onion powder

1 teaspoon paprika

1 teaspoon salt

⅛ teaspoon black pepper

Directions

Combine fish, spices, and lemon juice. Roll one small handful of mixture in a ball and flatten into patty. Grill on grill pan or broil, 4 minutes on each side.

Per serving: Calories 165.6; Fat 7.2 g (Saturated 1.1 g); Cholesterol 62.7 mg; Sodium 340.7 mg; Carbohydrate 1.0 g; Fiber 0.2 g; Protein 22.7 g

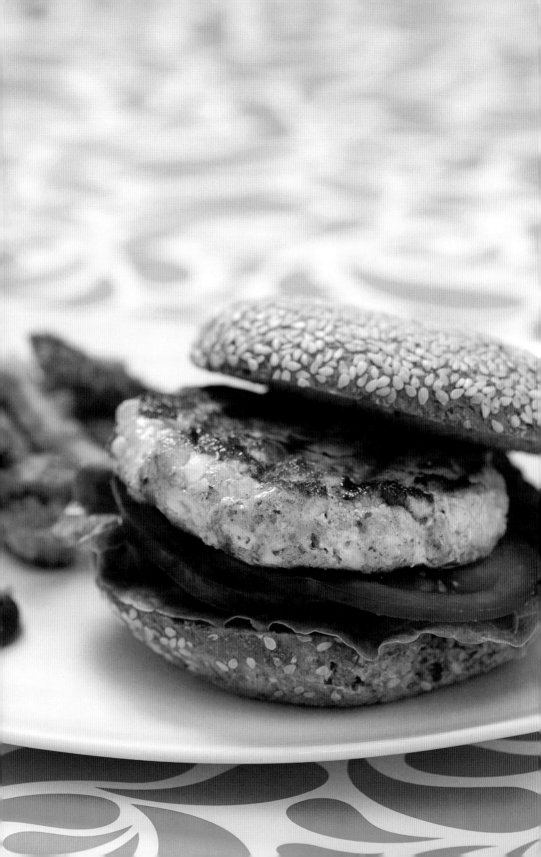

MINI FISH STICKS WITH HOMEMADE TARTAR DIPPING SAUCE

• • • • • • • • • • • • • • • • • • •

Serves 10

Ingredients

Mini Fish Sticks

1 tablespoon 1% reduced-fat milk

2 large eggs, lightly beaten

1 pound halibut fillets, cut into 20 (1-inch) strips

1 cup whole-grain panko (e.g., Ian's® Japanese breadcrumbs)

¼ cup flaxmeal

⅜ teaspoon kosher salt, divided

⅜ teaspoon freshly ground black pepper, divided

⅜ teaspoon garlic powder

⅜ teaspoon onion powder

2 tablespoon canola oil, divided

Dipping Sauce

¼ cup light sour cream

3 tablespoons canola mayonnaise

2 tablespoons bread-and-butter pickles, finely chopped

2 teaspoons capers, minced

Directions

Combine milk and eggs in a large bowl; stir with a whisk. Add fish and toss gently to coat. Place flaxmeal, panko, ¼ teaspoon salt, and ¼ teaspoon pepper in a large zip-top bag. Add fish to panko mixture; seal bag. Shake bag gently to coat fish.

Heat a large nonstick skillet over medium-high heat. Add 1 tablespoon oil to pan; swirl to coat. Add half of fish; cook 4 minutes or until done, turning occasionally to brown all sides. Repeat procedure with remaining 1 tablespoon oil and remaining fish.

In the meantime, combine sour cream, mayonnaise, pickles, capers, ⅛ teaspoon salt, and ⅛ teaspoon pepper in a small bowl for tartar dipping sauce. Serve sauce with fish.

Per serving (fish sticks): Calories 143.5; Fat 6.0 g (Saturated 0.7 g); Cholesterol 56.7 mg; Sodium 68.8 mg; Carbohydrate 5.8 g; Fiber 1.6 g; Protein 15.2 g

Per serving (sauce): Calories 31.5; Fat 2.3 g (Saturated 0.5 g); Cholesterol 2.5 mg; Sodium 98.7 mg; Carbohydrate 1.7 g; Fiber 0.0g; Protein 0.5 g

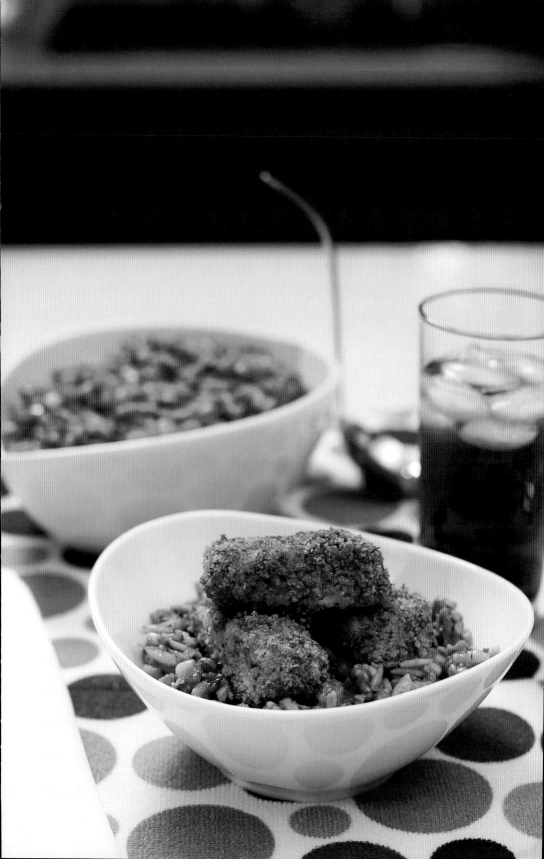

ARTICHOKE GIBBON

• •

Serves 8

Ingredients

1 small onion, finely chopped

2 garlic cloves, minced

2 teaspoons olive oil

2 whole eggs and 2 egg whites

¼ cup whole-wheat matzo meal

2 tablespoons minced fresh parsley

¼ teaspoon salt

⅛ teaspoon dried oregano

⅛ teaspoon pepper

6 ounces part-skim mozzarella cheese

½ cup cottage cheese

1 - 14-ounce can of water-packed
   artichoke hearts, rinsed,
   drained and chopped

Directions

Sauté onion and garlic in oil until tender; set aside. In a large bowl, whisk the eggs, matzo meal, parsley, salt, oregano, and pepper.

Stir in cheese, artichokes, and onion mixture. Pour into a greased nine-inch pie plate.* Bake at 350° F for 22–26 minutes or until a knife inserted near the center comes out clean.

*You can also put mixture into 100 percent whole-wheat pie shell or in mini cupcake holders and then bake.

Per serving: Calories 129.4; Fat 5.9 g (Saturated 2.8 g); Cholesterol 54.5 mg; Sodium 269.9 mg; Carbohydrate 8.7 g; Fiber 2.1 g; Protein 11.0 g

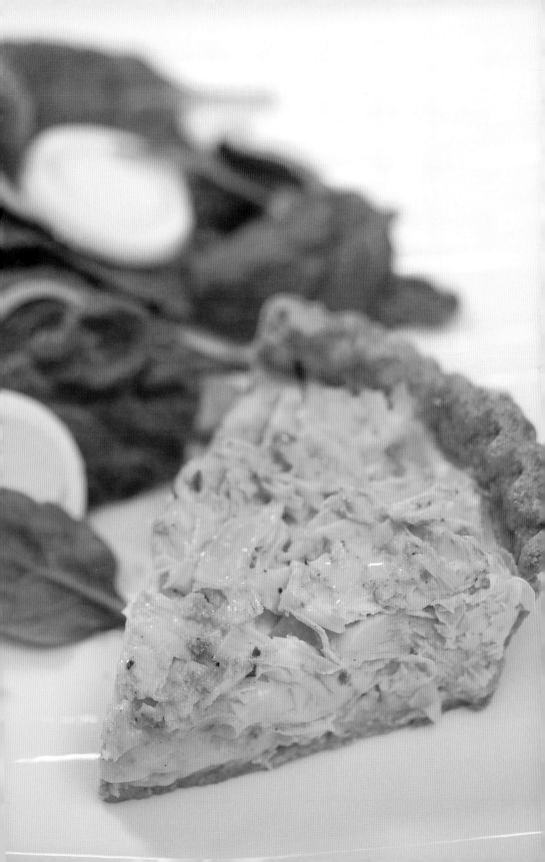

CHICKEN AND OKRA

* *

Serves 8

Ingredients

1 whole organic chicken,
    cut into 8 pieces

1 teaspoon paprika

1 teaspoon salt

1 teaspoon pepper

1 teaspoon garlic powder

2 teaspoons cinnamon,
    separated

1 tablespoon oil

4 tablespoons water

1–2 packages baby okra*

1 small can tomato paste (6 oz.)

Directions

Wash and clean the chicken. Place chicken pieces at the bottom of a small roaster. In a small bowl, combine the spices and oil. Brush the spice mixture around the pieces of chicken. Add 4 tablespoons of water to the roaster. Cover and bake at 350°F for 45 minutes. Take the roaster out of the oven and place the chicken pieces on a glass plate. Add in 1–2 packages of baby okra, fresh or frozen, into the chicken juices. Mix in 1 small can of tomato paste. Add the chicken back to the roaster and embed the pieces within the okra. Bake for 1 hour at 350° F.

    *You can also substitute the okra with Yukon potatoes, cubed, which would count towards the starch portion of your plate. The recipe contains meat.

Per serving: **Calories 144; Fat 4.7 g (Saturated 1.0 g); Cholesterol 63.4 mg; Sodium** 355.9 mg; Carbohydrate 2.7 g; Fiber 1.5 g; Protein 21.7 g

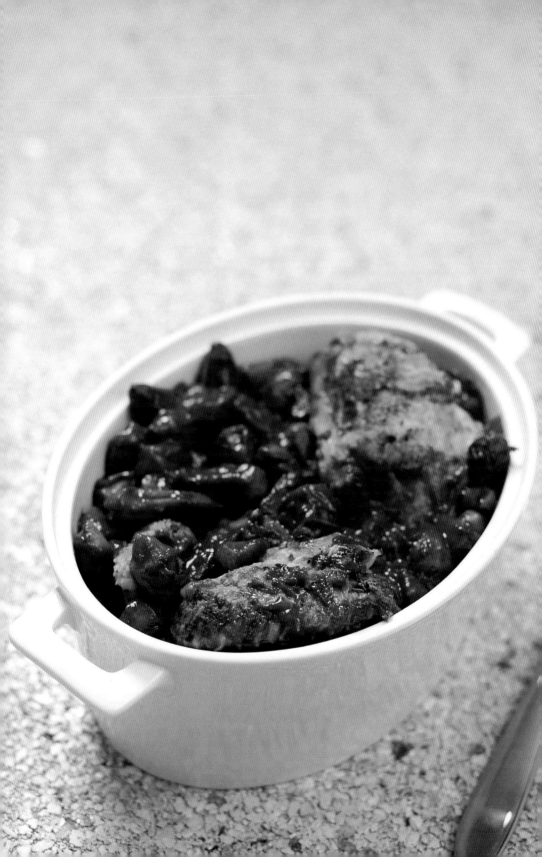

FASULIA—GREAT NORTHERN BEANS WITH MARROW BONES AND MEAT

● ● ● ● ● ● ● ● ● ● ● ● ● ● ● ● ● ● ●

Serves 8–10

Ingredients

2 garlic cloves, chopped

1 onion, chopped

2 tablespoons canola oil

1 pound flanken or beef chuck, cut in 2-inch cubes

OR 3 beef marrow bones

1 cup dried Great Northern Beans, soaked overnight in refrigerator and drained

2 tablespoons tomato paste

½ teaspoon ground cinnamon

¾ teaspoon kosher salt

Directions

Sauté garlic and onion in canola oil over medium heat about 4–6 minutes, or until onions are translucent. Add the meat and bones. Brown the meat. Add 2 quarts of water to the saucepan. Reduce the heat to low and simmer, uncovered, for 1 hour or until the meat is tender. Skim off any foam that rises to the top.

Add the beans, tomato paste, cinnamon, and salt and raise the heat to medium-high and bring to a boil. Reduce the heat to low and simmer, covered, for 2 hours. Cook longer if a thicker consistency is desired.

Per serving: Calories 194.8; Fat 9.6 g (Saturated 2.2 g); Cholesterol 49.1 mg; Sodium 312.1 mg; Carbohydrate 9.0 g; Fiber 2.7 g; Protein 17.5 g

Adapted from: Aromas of Aleppo.

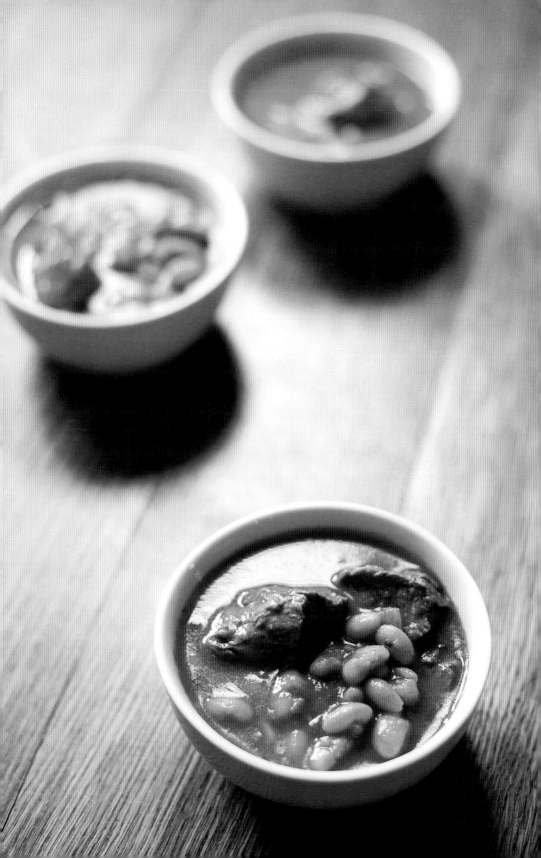

The next two dishes, Chamin and Moroccan fish, are traditional Moroccan recipes I learned from my husband's family. When I tried to get the recipes from my mother-in-law, Rebecca, and Tati (Grandma Susan), it was difficult to get serving sizes, as most dishes are adjusted to taste. I took a stab at writing them down, but you, too, may need to adjust for taste.

CHAMIN

● ● ● ● ● ● ● ● ● ● ● ● ● ● ● ● ● ● ● ●

Traditionally, chamin is cooked in a crockpot or a pot on the "blech" (hot plate) over Friday night and into the Sabbath day for lunch. A "complete meal," it is often served separated by the types of foods inside. It is best to begin preparing the different parts of the dish midday Friday or at least 2–3 hours before the Sabbath begins.

Ingredients

Serves 10

1 cup dried chickpeas

10 russet potatoes

2–4 whole eggs

1 pound of your choice of meat
　　(for example, "kichel")

1 teaspoon paprika

1 teaspoon all spice

1 teaspoon cumin

1 teaspoon extra virgin olive oil

Black pepper, to taste

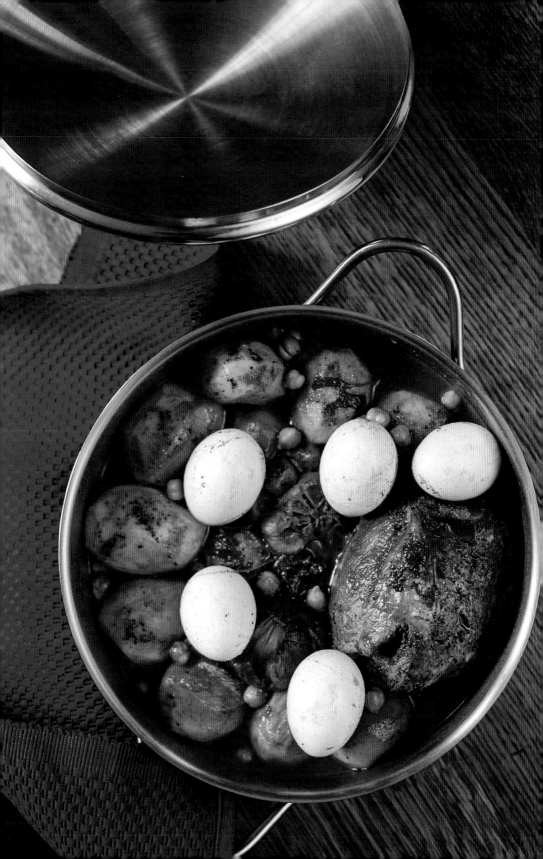

Directions

Prep the night before (for example, Thursday night, to begin cooking the chamin Friday, to be eaten Saturday). Soak ½ of fresh chickpeas in water. Clean about 10 russet potatoes and soak in water over night.

Cooking the dish on Friday:

In a large pot or crockpot, layer chickpeas (drained) on bottom, then potatoes, whole eggs (they cook inside the dish) and a piece of meat. Season with paprika, allspice, extra virgin olive oil, black pepper, and cumin. Cover with water. Simmer, boil, and cook through, 2–3 hours before Shabbat starts. Then cover the pot or crockpot and leave on "low" temperature until the Sabbath day meal on Saturday.

You may add a prune or date, without the pit, to the dish for sweetness and color; however, you should achieve a nice brown hue regardless because of the amount of spices used.

Per serving: Calories 167.9; Fat 11.2 g (Saturated 4.2 g); Cholesterol 71.2 mg; Sodium 115.5 mg; Carbohydrate 5.5 g; Fiber 1.1 g; Protein 10.5 g

MOROCCAN FISH

● ● ● ● ● ● ● ● ● ● ● ● ● ● ● ● ● ● ●

Serves 4

Ingredients

1 pound wild salmon

2 tomatoes, thinly sliced

7 whole garlic cloves

1 red pepper, thinly sliced in rounds

1 bunch cilantro, separated into two halves

2 tablespoons extra virgin olive oil, separated

1 tablespoon hot paprika or Israeli paprika

Salt and black pepper, to taste

1 lemon, thinly sliced, and lemon zest

1 jalapeño OR dried Chile OR dried sweet red pepper (hydrated in hot water a few minutes, then added to dish), optional

1 potato, sliced, optional

1 - 15-ounce can chickpeas, optional

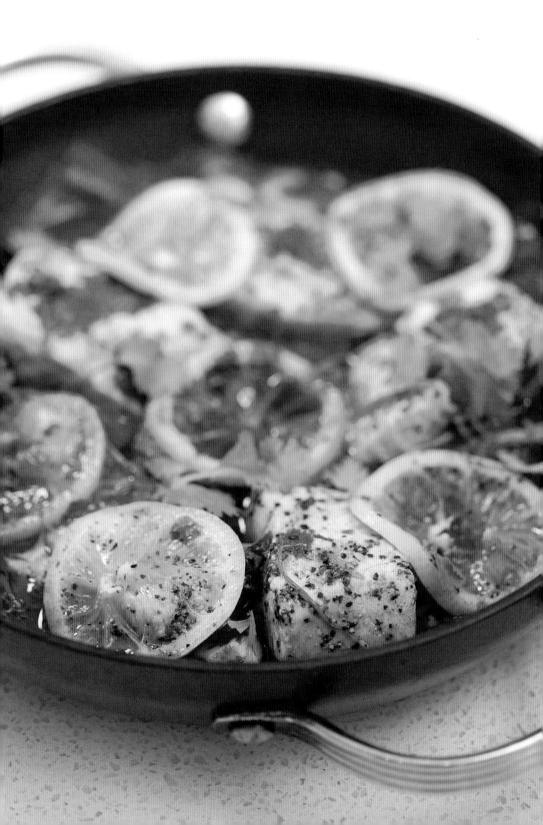

Directions

In a saucepan, layer tomatoes on the bottom of the pot. Then, layer red peppers on top of the tomatoes, followed by ½ the cilantro, then all the spices and fish on top. After that, season again with red pepper, salt, and black pepper. Drizzle 1 tablespoon of oil and layer the other ½ of chopped cilantro on top. Very thinly slice the lemon and grate its zest onto the top of the dish. If you want a more balanced meal, add sliced potato and/or a can of chickpeas to the dish. Cover and cook about 45 minutes over a medium flame, until the fish is cooked through.

Per serving: Calories 254.3; Fat 14.8 g (Saturated 2.2 g); Cholesterol 62.7; Sodium 59.3 mg; Carbohydrate 10.6 g; Fiber 3.5 g; Protein 24.4 g

SOUPS

HAMID (A TWIST ON VEGETABLE SOUP)

Serves 6

Ingredients

8 garlic cloves, peeled

1 small potato cut in 1-inch squares

2 celery stalks, diced

2 carrots, peeled and diced

Juice of 3 lemons

1 tablespoon dried mint leaves

1 teaspoon kosher salt

Directions

Smash garlic cloves with flat side of chef's knife. In medium saucepan, combine the garlic, potato, celery, carrots, lemon juice, mint, salt, and 5 cups water. Bring to a boil over medium heat. Reduce until vegetables are fork tender. Allow the broth to reduce to a thicker consistency.

Per serving: Calories 39.6; Fat 0.1 g (Saturated 0.0 g); Cholesterol 0.0 mg; Sodium 215.0 mg; Carbohydrate 10.0 g; Fiber 1.5 g; Protein 1.9 g

FENNEL SOUP

● ● ● ● ● ● ● ● ● ● ● ● ● ● ● ● ● ● ●

Serves 8

Adapted from cookinglight.com, this soup is a great way to get in your greens, without tasting too overbearing. To make it pareve, simply substitute the Greek yogurt with coconut milk.

Ingredients

2 red bell peppers

2 large fennel bulbs with stalks

2 tablespoons extra virgin olive oil

1 cup chopped shallots

1 tablespoon fresh thyme

⅜ teaspoon salt

4 cups water

2 cups organic no-chicken broth (e.g., Imagine Foods®)

1 bay leaf

4 ounces fresh spinach

¼ teaspoon freshly ground black pepper

½ cup fat-free Greek yogurt (to make recipe dairy)

OR ½ cup coconut milk (to make recipe pareve)

1 teaspoon grated lemon rind

1 teaspoon fresh lemon juice

Directions

Slice peppers in half, lengthwise. Discard seeds and membranes. Place pepper halves, skin side up, on foil-lined baking sheet. Broil 15 minutes or until blackened. Place in paper bag and fold to close tightly. Let stand for 10 minutes, then peel, chop, and set aside.

Cut fennel in half and discard core. Chop bulbs to measure one cup. Put fronds on side.

Heat oil in large saucepan. Add fennel, leek, shallots, thyme, and salt. Cover and cook 10 minutes stirring occasionally. Add broth, water, and bay leaf; bring to a boil. Cover, reduce heat, and simmer 12 minutes. Discard bay leaf. Stir in spinach and black pepper. Remove from heat; cover and let stand for 5 minutes. Use a hand blender and purée the soup.

Combine roasted bell peppers, yogurt or coconut milk, lemon rind, and lemon juice in food processor; process until smooth.

Serve ¾ cup soup in each bowl. Top with yogurt mixture and garnish with fennel fronds.

Per serving: Calories 92.7; Fat 3.8 g (Saturated 0.5 g); Cholesterol 0.0 mg; Sodium 195.3 mg; Carbohydrate 12.7 g; Fiber 3.1 g; Protein 3.6 g

STEFANIE'S CHICKEN SOUP

Serves 8

Ingredients

Broth

4 pieces organic chicken

1 quart water

10 baby carrots, diced

1 whole onion, peeled

½ green pepper

1 whole potato, peeled

2 celery stalks, diced

1 teaspoon parsley

1 tablespoon green dill

Salt and pepper, to taste

Matzo ball

4 pastured eggs

4 tablespoons cold water

4 tablespoons oil

1 cup whole-wheat matzo meal

1 teaspoon salt

1 teaspoon pepper

Directions

Put chicken in a large soup pot and cover with water. Boil for 1 hour. Combine all matzo ball ingredients and refrigerate mixture for at least 15 minutes.

Add all the remaining and spices to the boiling chicken soup. Boil about a half hour more and then form matzo balls and throw into the soup. Boil 10 minutes more.

Per serving: Calories 198.3; Fat 9.4 g (Saturated 1.3 g); Cholesterol 86.1 mg; Sodium 370.7 mg; Carbohydrate 21.9 g; Fiber 2.0 g; Protein 6.3 g

SHERRY'S LENTIL SOUP (ADES SOUP)

Serves 4

Ingredients

1 cup split red lentils

4 cups water

2 large cloves of garlic, crushed

½ teaspoon coriander

1 tablespoon coarse salt

2 tablespoons canola oil

Cumin and crushed red pepper,
to taste

Lemon juice, to taste, optional

Directions

Rinse lentils and add to water. Boil over low flame until creamy. Stir garlic with salt and coriander and sauté in oil. Add to lentils and simmer for 1 hour. Serve with taste of cumin and crushed red pepper and squeezed lemon if desired.

Per serving: Calories 59.7; Fat 0.2 g; (Saturated 0.0 g); Cholesterol 0.0 mg; Sodium 630.2 mg; Carbohydrate 10.5 g; Fiber 3.9 g; Protein 4.6 g

BREAKFASTS AND DESSERTS

SOURDOUGH FRENCH TOAST

● ●

Serves 4

Ingredients

8 slices whole-wheat sourdough
bread (e.g. Bread Alone)

1 egg

1 cup almond milk

1 teaspoon cinnamon

Directions

Whisk together almond milk, egg, and cinnamon. Drench bread in mixture. In a shallow frying pan, spray cooking spray and heat the pan. Add the bread and cook on each side for about 3 minutes, until browned.

Per serving: Calories 194.5; Fat 3.8 g (Saturated 0.4 g); Cholesterol 46.5 mg; Sodium 375.4 mg; Car; Fiber 4.6 g; Protein 7.8 g

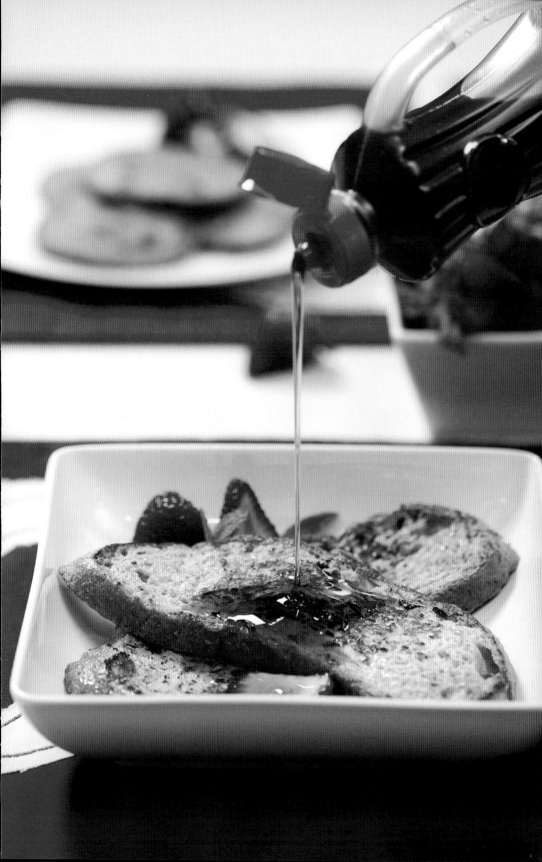

BUCKWHEAT PANCAKES

Serves 12

Ingredients

1 cup buckwheat flour

1 egg

1 cup almond milk

1 teaspoon almond extract

Directions

In a medium skillet, spray with non-stick cooking spray on medium flame. When hot, place ¼ cup mixture into the skillet. Cook pancake until bubbles begin to form on the top of the pancake, then flip. Cook for about 1–2 minutes more, until you can easily remove the pancake from the skillet. Repeat with the entire mixture.

Per serving: Calories 84.4; Fat 1.9 g (Saturated 0.3 g); Cholesterol 31.0 mg; Sodium 36.8 mg; Carbohydrate 13.5 g; Fiber 3.0 g; Protein 3.8 g

HOMEMADE NUTELLA

● ●

Serves 8

Ingredients

½ cup hazelnut butter* (or
  almond butter)
1–2 tablespoons unsweetened

cocoa powder
1–2 tablespoons raw honey or
  maple syrup

Directions

Place hazelnut butter in a shallow bowl. Add cocoa powder and mix it into the nut butter with a fork. Mix in honey or maple syrup. Taste and adjust seasonings. If you need to thin the mixture, add hazelnut oil, walnut oil, or coconut oil (warmed to liquid consistency).

*To make your own hazelnut butter, toast hazelnuts on a cookie sheet in a 400° F oven for about 10 minutes. Remove as much of the nut skins as possible in a damp towel, add to a food processor and process into a paste.

Adapted from: Realfoodkosher.com.

Per serving: Calories 105.2; Fat 8.8 g (Saturated 0.7 g); Cholesterol 0.0 mg; Sodium 2.0 mg; Carbohydrate 5.8 g; Fiber 1.8 g; Protein 2.5 g

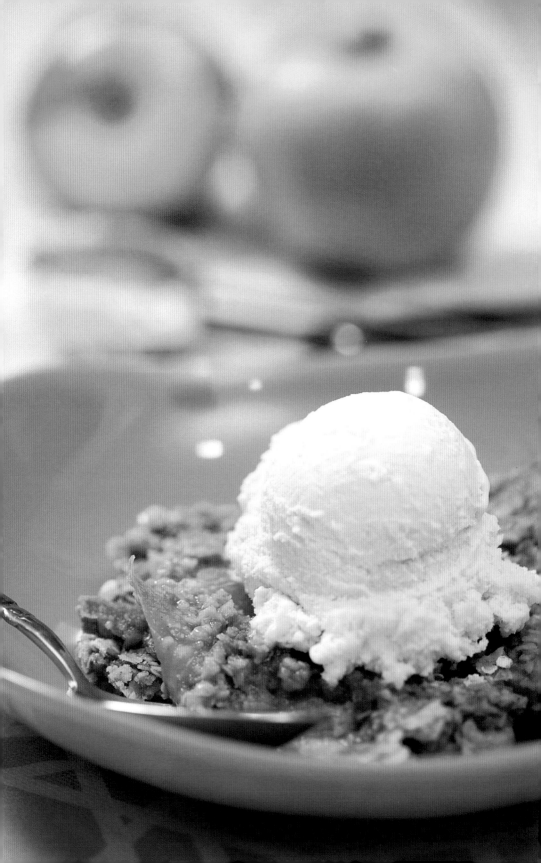

HEALTHY APPLE CRISP

● ●

Serves 6

Ingredients

4 medium tart apples, peeled and
   thinly sliced

⅓ cup whole-wheat pastry flour,
   divided

1 tablespoon honey

2 teaspoons lemon juice

¾ teaspoon ground cinnamon,
   divided

⅔ cup old-fashioned oats

½ cup agave syrup

1 tablespoon coconut spread

Organic vanilla coconut ice cream
   or almond milk ice cream,
   optional

Directions

In a large bowl, combine the apples, 1 tablespoon flour, honey, lemon juice, and ¼ teaspoon cinnamon. Pour into a greased 9-inch deep-dish pie plate.

In a small bowl, combine the oats, agave, and remaining flour and cinnamon. Cut in coconut spread until crumbly; sprinkle over apple mixture.

Cover with waxed paper. Microwave on high for 5–7 minutes or until apples are tender. Serve with ice cream, if desired.

Per serving (1 cup, without ice cream) Calories 212.5; Fat 6.3 g (Saturated 2.5 g); Cholesterol 0.0 mg; Sodium 39.1 mg; Carbohydrate 42.5 g; Fiber 5.3 g; Protein 1.8 g

Per serving (1 cup, with ice cream): Calories: 252; Fat: 7 g (4 g saturated fat); Cholesterol: 15 mg; Sodium: 66 mg; Carbohydrates: 49 g; Fiber: 3g; Protein: 2g.

POPCORN WITH DARK CHOCOLATE DRIZZLE

• •

Serves 6

Ingredients

½ cup organic popcorn kernels

1 tablespoon canola oil

1 teaspoon salt

2 ounces 70% dark chocolate

Directions

Coat the bottom of the pan with oil. Cover kernels in a single layer. Add salt. Cover pot. Put on medium flame. Turn off when there's a pause between popping. Close heat and allow continued popping with lid on. When complete, move popped corn to baking sheet and spread out.

Melt chocolate over hot water bath (see Banana with Dark Chocolate and Chopped Peanuts). Drizzle over popcorn. Allow to cool and harden.

Per serving Calories 83.8; Fat 5.5 g (Saturated 2.2 g); Cholesterol 1.3 mg; Sodium 391.5 mg; Carbohydrate 9.4 g; Fiber 1.4 g; Protein 1.0 g

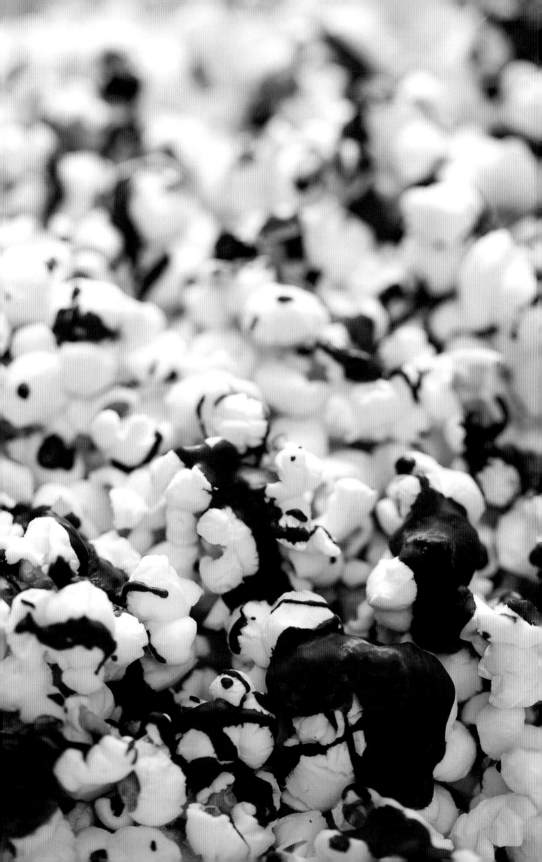

HUMMUS WITH PEANUT BUTTER

● ● ● ● ● ● ● ● ● ● ● ● ● ● ● ● ● ● ● ●

Serves 6

Ingredients

3 tablespoons natural creamy
   peanut butter

3 tablespoons fresh lemon juice

1 tablespoon plus 2 teaspoons
   olive oil

½ teaspoon ground cumin

½ teaspoon black pepper

⅜ teaspoon kosher salt

1 - 15½-ounce can chickpeas,
   rinsed and drained

1 garlic clove, minced

7 tablespoons water

4 Persian cucumbers cut into
   ¼-inch-thick slices

Directions

Combine peanut butter and next seven ingredients (through garlic) in a food processor. With food processor running, slowly drizzle in water; process until smooth. Serve with cucumber as mini sandwiches (hummus in between). Roll in black or white sesame seeds, if desired.

Per serving: Calories 148.2; Fat 6.6 g (Saturated 1.0 g); Cholesterol 0.0 mg; Sodium 288.1 mg; Carbohydrate 18.8 g; Fiber 4.1 g; Protein 5.0 g

NOTES

[1] *Cooley's Cyclopaedia of Practical Receipts*, 6th ed. (1880)

[2] B. Wansink and KV Ittersum. "Portion Size Me: Downsizing our Consumption Norms." *Journal of the American Dietetic Association* (2007): 1–4.

[3] Babylonian Talmud, Gittin 70a

[4] J. Slavin. "Dietary Fiber and Body Weight." *Nutrition* 21 (2005): 411–18.

[5] S. Woods. "Gastrointestinal Satiety Signals I. An Overview of Gastrointestinal Signals that Influence Food Intake." *American Journal of Physiology* 286 (2004): G7–G13.

[6] J. Broussard, D. Ehrmann, E. Cauter, E. Tasali, M. Brady. "Impaired Insulin Signaling in Human Adipocytes After Experimental Sleep Restriction: A Randomized, Crossover Study." *Annal of Internal Medicine.* 157 (2012): 549–557.

[7] F. McKiernan, et. al. "Relationships between human thirst, hunger, drinking, and feeding." *Physiology & Behavior* 94 (2008): 700–08.

[8] A. Kant, B. Graubard, E. Atchison. "Intakes of plain water, moisture in foods and beverages, and total water in the adult US population—nutritional, meal pattern, and body weight correlates. National Health and Nutrition Examination Surveys 1999–2006." *American Journal of Clinical Nutrition* 90 (2009): 655–663.

[9] Rav Chisda. Talmud. Berochot 40A.

[10] IOM: http://www.iom.edu/Global/News%20Announcements/~/media/442A08B899 F44DF9AAD083D86164C75B.ashx

[11] W. C. Willet, et al. "Coffee Consumption and Coronary Heart Disease in Women. A Ten-Year Follow-up." *Journal of the American Medical Association* 275 (1996): 458–62.

[12] M. Leone, D. Zhai, S. Sareth, S. Kitada, J.C. Reed, M. Pellecchia. "Cancer prevention by tea polyphenols is linked to their direct inhibition of antiapoptotic Bcl-2-family proteins". *Cancer Research* 63 (2003): 8118–21.

[13] A.M. Hill, et al. "Can EGCG Reduce Abdominal Fat in Obese Subjects?" *Journal of the American College of Nutrition* 26 (2007): 396S–402S.

[14] S. Malik, D.S. Mohar. "The Sirtuin System: The Holy Grail of Resveratrol?" *Journal of Clinical & Experimental Cardiology* 3 (2012): 216.

[15] Ramabam. Laws of Understanding. Chapter 5, Law 3.

[16] M. Bes-rastrollo, N. Wedick, M. Martinez-Gonzalex, T. Li, L. Sampson, F. Hu. "Prospective study of nut consumption, long-term weight change, and obesity risk in women." *American Journal of Clinical Nutrition* 89 (2009): 1913–1919.

[17] G.D. Foster, P.M. Kris-Etherton, R.D. Mattes. "Impact of peanuts and tree nuts on body weight and healthy weight loss in adults." *Journal of Nutrition* 138 (2008) 1741S–1745S.

[18] C. Colantuoni, P. Rada, J. McCarthy, C. Patten, N.M. Avena, A.N. Chadeayne, B.G. Hoebel. "Evidence that intermittent, excessive sugar intake causes endogenous opiod dependence." *Obesity Research* 10 (2012): 478–488.

[19] J.A. Cocores, M.S. Gold. "The salted food addiction hypothesis may explain overeating and the obesity epidemic." *Medical Hypothesis* 73 (2009) 892–9.

[20] J.R. Ifland, H.G. Preuss, M.T. Marcus, K.M. Rourke, et al. "Refined food addiction: A classic substance use disorder." *Medical Hypothesis* 72 (2009): 518–526.

[21] A. Paoli, G. Marcolin, F. Zonin, M. Neri, A. Sivieri, Q.F. Pacelli. "Exercising fasting or fed to enhance fat loss? Influence of food intake on respiratory ratio and excess postexercise oxygen consumption after a bout of endurance training." *International Journal of Sport Nutrition and Exercise Metabolism* 21 (2011): 48–54.

[22] C. C. Gómez, L. M. Bermejo, K. V. Loria. "Importance of a balanced Omega 6/Omega 3 ratio for the maintenance of health. Nutritional recommendations." *Nutricion Hospitalaria* 25 (2011): 323–9.

[23] T. Mickleborough."Omega-3 Polyunsaturated Fatty Acids in Physical Performance Optimization." *International Journal of Sport Nutrition & Exercise Metabolism* 23 (2013): 83–96.

[24] G. Combs. *The Vitamins.* (Waltham, Massachusetts: Academic Press, 2012).

[25] A. Drewnowski, E. Almiron-Roig, "Human Perceptions and Preferences for Fat-Rich Foods," in *Fat Detection: Taste, Texture, and Post Ingestive Effects*, eds. J. P. Montmayeur, J. le Coutre (Boca Raton: CRC Press, 2010).

[26] E. Rolls. "Taste, olfactory, and food texture processing in the brain, and the control of food intake." *Physiology & Behavior* 19 (2005): 45–56.

[27] G.J. Schwartz, J. Fu, G. Astarita, X. Li, S. Gaetani, P. Campolongo, V. Cuomo, D Piomelli. "The lipid messenger OEA links dietary fat intake to satiety." Cell Metabolism 8 (2008): 281–8.

[28] C. Strik, F. Lithander, A.T. McGill, A. MacGibbon, B. McArdle, S. Popitto. "No evidence of differential effects of SFA, MUFA or PUFA on post-ingestive satiety and energy intake: a randomised trial of fatty acid saturation." *Nutrition Journal* 9 (2010): 24.

[29] S. Matsumura, A. Eguchi, Y. Okafuji, S. Tatsu, T. Mizushige, S. Tsuzuki, K. Inoue, T. Fushiki. "Dietary fat ingestion activates β-endorphin neurons in the hypothalamus." *FEBS Lett* 586 (2012): 1231–5.

[30] Martin, CK, Rosenbaum, D, Han, H, Geiselman, P, et al. Change in food cravings, food preferences, and appetite during a low-carbohydrate and low-fat diet. *Obesity* 201; 19: 1963–1970.

[31] J. L. Martineau. "Free fatty acid availability and temperature regulation in cold water." Journal of Applied Physiology 67(1989): 2466–72.

[32] A.C. Logan. "Omega-3 fatty acids and major depression: A primer for the mental health professional." *Lipids in Health and Disease* 3 (2004): 25.

[33] M. Maes, A. Christophe, J. Delanghe, C. Altamura, H. Neels, H.Y. Meltzer."Lowered Omega3 polyunsaturated fatty acids in serum phospholipids and cholesteryl esters of depressed patients." Psychiatric Research 85 (1999): 275–291.

[34] H. Tiemeier, H. R. van Tuijl, A. Hofman, A.J. Kiliaan, M.M. Breteler. "Plasma fatty acid composition and depression are associated in the elderly: the Rotterdam Study." *American Journal of Clinical Nutrition* 78 (2003): 40–6.

[35] V. Danthiir, N.R. Burns, T. Nettelbeck, C. Wilson, G. Wittert. "The older people, Omega-3, and cognitive health (EPOCH) trial design and methodology: A randomised, double-blind, controlled trial investigating the effect of long-chain Omega-3 fatty acids on cognitive ageing and wellbeing in cognitively healthy older adults." *Nutrition Journal* 10 (2011): 117.

[36] J.E. Karr, J.E. Alexander, R.G. Winningham. "Omega-3 polyunsaturated fatty acids and cognition throughout the lifespan: a review." *Nutritional Neuroscience* 14 (2011): 216–25.

[37] Mayo Clinic. "Omega-3 fatty acids, fish oil, alpha-linolenic acid." (Accessed: 6/18/13) http://www.mayoclinic.com/health/fish-oil/NS_patient-fishoil/DSECTION=evidence

American Optometric Association. "Essential Fatty Acids." American Optometric Association Website (Accessed: 6/18/13) http://www.aoa.org/x11853.xml

N.G. Bazan, M.F. Molina, W.C. Gordon. "Docosahexaenoic Acid Signalolipidomics in Nutrition: Significance in Aging, Neuroinflammation, Macular Degeneration, Alzheimer's, and Other Neurodegenerative Diseases." *Annual* 31 (2011): 321–351.

38 R. Wander, "A Primer on Dietary Fat: The Good, the Bad and the Unknown." Linus Pauling Institute (Accessed: 6/18/13) http://lpi.oregonstate.edu/f-w98/primer.html

39 S. Egert, M. Kratz, F. Kannenberg, M. Fobker, U. Wahrburg. "Effects of high-fat and low-fat diets rich in monounsaturated fatty acids on serum lipids, LDL size and indices of lipid peroxidation in healthy non-obese men and women when consumed under controlled conditions." *European Journal of Nutrition* 50 (2011): 71–9.

40 P.V. Johnston, F.A. Kummerow, C.H. Walton. "Origin of the trans fatty acids in human tissue." Experimental Biology and Medicine 99, no. 3 (1958): 735–6.

41 A. Ascherio, C.H. Hennekens, J.E. Buring, C. Master, M.J. Stampfer, W.C. Willett. "Trans-fatty acids intake and risk of myocardial infarction." *Circulation* 89 (1994): 94–101.

42 W.C. Willett, M.J. Stampfer, J.E. Manson, et al. "Intake of trans fatty acids and risk of coronary heart disease among women." *Lancet* 341 (1993): 581–5.

43 M.B. Katan, P.L. Zock, R.P. Mensink. "Trans fatty acids and their effects on lipoproteins in humans." *Annual Review of Nutrition* 15 (1995): 473–93.

44 C. Degen, J. Ecker, S. Piegholdt, G. Liebisch, G. Schmitz, G. Jahreis. "Metabolic and growth inhibitory effects of conjugated fatty acids in the cell line HT-29 with special regard to the conversion of t11,t13-CLA." *BBA-Molecular & Cell Biology of Lipids* 1811 (2011): 1070–80.

45 A.P. Nugent, H.M. Roche, E.J. Noone, A. Long, D.K. Kelleher, M.J. Gibney. "The effects of conjugated linoleic acid supplementation on immune function in healthy volunteers." *European Journal of Clinical Nutrition* 59 (2005): 742–50.

46 L.D. Whigham, A.C. Watras, D.A. Schoeller. "Efficacy of conjugated linoleic acid for reducing fat mass: a meta-analysis in humans." *American Journal of Clinical Nutrition* 85 (2007): 1203–11.

47 F. Moloney, T.P. Yeow, A. Mullen, J.J. Nolan, H.M. Roche. "Conjugated linoleic acid supplementation, insulin sensitivity, and lipoprotein metabolism in patients with type 2 diabetes mellitus." *American Journal of Clinical Nutrition* 80 (2004): 887–95.

48 D.E. Butz, L. Guangmin, S.M. Huebner, M.E. Cook. "A mechanistic approach to understanding conjugated linoleic acid's role in inflammation using murine models of rheumatoid arthritis." *American Journal of Physiology* 293 (2007): R669–R676.

49 N. Aryaeian, F. Shahram, M. Djalali, M.R. Eshragian, A. Djazayeri, A. Sarrafnejad, A. Salimzadeh, N. Naderi, C. Maryam. "Effect of conjugated linoleic acids,

vitamin E and their combination on the clinical outcome of Iranian adults with active rheumatoid arthritis." International Journal of Rheumatic Disease12 (2009): 20–8.

50 L.G. Funck, D. Barrera-Arellano, J.M. Block. "Conjugated linoleic acid (CLA) and its relationship with cardiovascular disease and associated risk factors." *Archivos Latinoamericanos de Nutr*icion 56 (2006): 123–34.

51 H.B. MacDonald. "Conjugated Linoleic Acid and Disease Prevention: A Review of Current Knowledge." *Journal of the American College of Nutrition* 2 (2000): 111S–118S.

52 K.W. Lee, H.J. Lee, H.Y. Cho, Y.J. Kim. "Role of the conjugated linoleic acid in the prevention of cancer." *Critical Review in Food Science Nutr*ition 45 (2005): 135–44.

N.S. Kelley, N.E. Hubbard, K.L. Erickson. "Conjugated Linoleic Acid Isomers and Cancer." *Journal of Nutrition.* 137 (2007): 2599–2607.

53 J.M. Gaullier, J. Halse, K. Høye, K. Kristiansen, H. Fagertun, H. Vik, O. Gudmund-sen. "Conjugated linoleic acid supplementation for 1 y reduces body fat mass in healthy overweight humans." *American Journal of Clinical Nutrition* 79 (2004): 1118–25.

54 G.D. Lawrence. "Dietary fats and health: Dietary recommendations in the context of scientific evidence." *Advances in Nutrition* 4 (2013): 294–302.

55 M. Enig, "The Importance of Saturated Fats for Biological Functions." Westin A. Price Foundation (2004). http://www.westonaprice.org/know-your-fats/importance-of-saturated-fats-for-biological-functions

56 A.B. Feranil, P.L. Duazo, C.W. Kuzawa, L.S. Adair. "Coconut oil is associated with a beneficial lipid profile in pre-menopausal women in the Philippines." *Asia Pacific Journal of Clinical Nutrition* 20 (2011): 190–5.

57 R. Micha, D. Mozaffarian. "Saturated Fat and Cardiometabolic Risk Factors, Coronary Heart Disease, Stroke, and Diabetes: a Fresh Look at the Evidence." *Lipids* (2010): 893–905.

58 Babylonian Talmud, Tractate Pesachim: 42.

59 A.J. Richardson. "Omega-3 fatty acids in ADHD and related neurodevelopmental disorders." *International Review of Psychiatry* 18 (2006): 155–72.

60 M.H. Block, A. Qawasmi. "Omega-3 fatty acid supplementation for the treatment of children with attention-deficit/hyperactivity disorder symptomatology: Systematic review and meta-analysis." *Journal of the American Academy of Child & Adolescent Psychiatry* 50 (2011): 991–1000.

61 A.P. Simopoulos. "The importance of the ratio of Omega-6/Omega-3 essential fatty acids." *Biomedicine & Pharmacotherapy* 56 (2002): 365–79.

62 C. Ramsden, D. Zamora, L. Boonseng, et al. "Use of dietary linoleic acid for secondary prevention of coronary heart disease and death: evaluation of recovered data from the Sydney Diet Heart Study and updated meta-analysis." *BMJ* 346 (2013): e8707.

63 D. Swanson, R. Block, S.A. Mousa. "Omega-3 fatty acids EPA and DHA: health benefits throughout life." *Advances in Nutrition* 3 (2012): 1–7.

64 R. Estruch, E. Ros, J. Salas-Salvadó, et al. "Primary prevention of cardiovascular disease with a Mediterranean diet." *New England Journal of Medicine* (Accessed 3/6/2013) http://www.nejm.org/doi/full/10.1056/NEJMoa1200303.

65 F.B. Hu, M.J. Stampfer, J.E. Manson, et al. "Frequent nut consumption and risk of coronary heart disease in women: prospective cohort study." *BMJ* 7169, no. 317 (1998): 1341–45.

66 T. Hyun, E. Barrett-Connor, D. Milne. "Zinc intakes and plasma concentrations in men with osteoporosis: the Rancho Bernardo Study." *American Journal of Clinical Nutrition* 80, no. 3 (2004): 715–721.

67 J. Vinson, Y. Cai. "Nuts, especially walnuts, have both antioxidant quantity and efficacy and exhibit significant potential health benefits." *Food & Function* 3 (2012): 134–40.

68 M. Guevara-Cruz, A. R. Tovar, C. Aguilar-Salinas, I. Medina-Vera, L. Gil-Zenteno, I. Hernández-Viveros, N. Torres. "A dietary pattern including nopal, chia seed, soy protein, and oat reduces serum triglycerides and glucose intolerance in patients with metabolic Syndrome1-4." *The Journal of Nutrition* 142 (2013): 64–9.

G. I. Travis, C. C. Jason, A. B. Phillip. "Omega-3 chia seed loading as a means of carbohydrate loading." *Journal of Strength and Conditioning Research* 25 (2011): 61–65.

B.M. Ross, J. Seguin, L.E. Sieswerda. "Omega-3 fatty acids as treatments for mental illness: which disorder and which fatty acid?" *Lipids in Health & Disease* (2007): 621–39. doi:10.1186/1476-511X-6-21.

69 Mishneh Torah, Ma'achalot Assurot 9:28.

70 T. Karapinar, M. Dabak, O. Kizil. "Thiamine status of feedlot cattle fed a high-concentrate diet." *Canadian Vet Journal* (2010): 1251–3.

71 C.A. Daley, A. Abbott, S. Larson, et. al. "A review of fatty acid profiles and antioxidant content in grass-fed and grain-fed beef." *Nutrition Journal* 9 (2010): 10.

72 S. K. Duckett, et al. "Effects of winter stocker growth rate and finishing system on: III. Tissue proximate, fatty acid, vitamin, and cholesterol content." *Journal of Animal Science* (2009). doi: 10.2527/jas.2009-1850.

[73] L. Ellis, "Preventing Dementia Risk." Aetna (2003). http://www intelihealth.com/ IH/ihtIH/WSANP000/325/28910/328885.html?d=dmtContent

[74] R. De Giorgio, G. Barbara. "Is irritable bowel syndrome an inflammatory disorder?" *Current Gastroenterology Reports*. 4, no. 10 (2008): 385–90.

O. A. Ashaye, L. B. Taiwo, S. B. Fasoyiro, C. A. Akinnagbe. "Compositional and shelf-life properties of soy-yogurt using two starter cultures." *Nutrition and Food Science* 31 (2001): 247–250.

A. Kebede, B. C. Viljoen, T. H. Gadaga, J. A. Narvhus, A. Lourens-Hattingh. "The effect of container type on the growth of yeast and lactic acid bacteria during production of Sethemi, South African spontaneously fermented milk." *Food Research International* 40, no. 1 (2007): 33–38.

[75] C. G. Prosser CG, R. D. Mclaren, D. Frost, M. Agnew, D.J. Lowry. "Composition of the non-protein nitrogen fraction of goat whole milk powder and goat milk-based infant and follow-on formulae." *International Journal of Food Sciences and Nutrition* 59, no. 2 (2008): 123–33.

Daddaoua, et. al. "Goat Milk Oligosaccharides Are Anti-Inflammatory in Rats with Hapten-Induced Colitis." *Journal of Nutrition* 136 (2006): 672–6.

[76] E. I. El-Agamy. "The challenge of cow milk protein allergy." *Small Ruminant Research* 68, no. 1 (2007): 64–72.

[77] G. Freund. "Use of goat milk for infant feeding: experimental work at Créteil (France). (Proceeding of the meeting *Intérêts nutritionnel et diététique du lait de chèvre*." (Niort, France: INRA, 1996):119–21.

[78] O. Razafindrakoto, N. Ravelomanana, A. Rasolofo, R.D. Rakotoarimanana, P. Gourgue, P. Coquin, A. Briend. "Goat's milk as a substitute for cow's milk in undernourished children: a randomized double-blind clinical trial." *Pediatrics* 94, no. 1 (1994): 65–9.

Y. W. Park, M. Juárez, M. Ramos, G. F. W. Haenlein. "Physico-chemical characteristics of goat and sheep milk." *Small Ruminant Research* 68, no. 1 (2007): 88–113.

[79] M. Mihoc, G. Pop, E. Alexa, I. Radulov. "Nutritive quality of Romanian hemp varieties (Cannabis sativa L.) with special focus on oil and metal contents of seeds." *Chemistry Central Journal* 6 (2012): 122.

[80] G. Combs. *The Vitamins*. (Waltham, Massachusetts: Academic Press, 2012).

[81] A. Sapone, J. Bai, C. Ciacci, et. al. "Spectrum of gluten-related disorders: consensus on new nomenclature and classification." *BMC Medicine* 10 (2012): 13.

[82] S. Boyles. "Gluten Sensitivity: Fact or Fad?" WEBMD (Accessed: 6/20/13). http://www.webmd.com/diet/news/20120220/gluten-sensitivity-fact-or-fad

[83] K. O'Brien. "Should We All Go Gluten Free?" The New York Times Online. (Accessed: 6/20/2013). http://www.nytimes.com/2011/11/27/magazine/Should-We-All-Go-Gluten-Free.html?pagewanted=all&_r=0

[84] H. Xu, G.T. Barnes, Q. Yang, et al. "Chronic inflammation in fat plays a crucial role in the development of obesity-related insulin resistance." *Journal of Clinical Investigation* 112 (2003): 1821–1830.

[85] F. Soares, R. Oliveira Matoso, L. Teixeira, et al. "Gluten-free diet reduces adiposity, inflammation and insulin resistance associated with the induction of PPAR-alpha and PPAR-gamma expression." *The Journal of Nutritional Biochemistry* 24 (2012): 1105–1111.

[86] E. D. Newnham. "Does gluten cause gastrointestinal symptoms in subjects without coeliac disease?" *Journal of Gastroenterology and Hepatology Supplement* 3 (2011): 132–134.

J. R. Biesiekierski, E. D. Newnham, P. M. Irving, et al. "Gluten causes gastrointestinal symptoms in subjects without celiac disease: a double-blind randomized placebo-controlled trial." *American Journal of Gastroenterology* 106 (2011): 508–514.

A. Carroccio, I. Brusca, P. Mansueto, et al. "A cytologic assay for diagnosis of food hypersensitivity in patients with irritable bowel syndrome." *Clinical Gastroenterology & Hepatology* 8 (2010): 254–260.

A. Fasano, et al. "Prevalence of celiac disease in at-risk and not-at-risk groups in the United States: a large multicenter study." *Archives of Internal Medicine* 163 (2003): 286–92.

[87] A. Carroccio, I. Brusca, P. Mansueto, et al. "A cytologic assay for diagnosis of food hypersensitivity in patients with irritable bowel syndrome." *Clinical Gastroenterology & Hepatology* 8, no. 3 (2010): 254–260.

[88] R.S. Gibson, K. B. Bailey, M. Gibbs, E. L. Ferguson. "A review of phytate, iron, zinc, and calcium concentrations in plant-based complementary foods used in low-income countries and implications for bioavailability." *Food and Nutrition Bulletin* 31 (2010): S134–46.

[89] L. Bohn, A. Meyer, S. Rasussen. "Phytate: impact on environment and human nutrition. A challenge for molecular breeding." *Journal of Zhejiang University Science* 9, no. 3 (2008): 165–191.

[90] Hemalatha S, Platel, K, Srinivasan, K. "Influence of germination and fermentation on bioaccessibility of zinc and iron from food grains." *European Journal of Clinical Nutrition* 61, no. 3 (2007): 342–8.

[91] "Stamped Product List." Whole Grain Council Website. (2013) http://wholegrains-council.org/find-whole-grains/stamped-products

[92] M. Gibney, H. Voster, F. Kok. *Introduction to Human Nutrition* (Hoboken: Wiley-Blackwell, 2012).

[93] M. Lenoir, F. Serre, L. Cantin, S. H. Ahmed. "Intense Sweetness Surpasses Cocaine Reward." *PLoS ONE* 8, no 2. (2007): e698.

[94] "Carbohydrates: Good Carbs Guide the Way." Harvard School of Public Health. (Accessed: 6/20/2013). http://www.hsph.harvard.edu/nutritionsource/carbohydrates-full-story/

[95] L. Morenga, M. Levers, S. Williams, R. Brown, J. Mann. "Comparison of high protein and high fiber weight-loss diets in women with risk factors for the metabolic syndrome: a randomized trial." *Nutrition Journal* 10 (2011): 40.

[96] E. A. Knut, A. Alaedini, et al. "Non-celiac gluten sensitivity." *Gastrointestinal Endoscopy Clinics of North America* 22 (2012): 723–734.

[97] J. R. Biesiekierski, E. D. Newnham, P.M. Irving, et al. "Gluten causes gastrointestinal symptoms in subjects without celiac disease: a double-blind randomized placebo-controlled trial." *American Journal of Gastroenterology* 106 (2011): 508–514. Abstract.

[98] K. O'Brien. "Should we all go gluten-free?" The New York Times Online (Accessed: 01/25/13.) http://www.nytimes.com/2011/11/27/magazine/Should-We-All-Go-Gluten-Free.html?pagewanted=all&_r=0
Abstract I Arch 2003 Feb 10;163(3):286-92.

[99] H.C. Hung, K. J. Joshipura, R. Jiang, et al. "Fruit and vegetable intake and risk of major chronic disease." *Journal of the National Cancer Institute* 96 (2004): 1577–84.

[100] F. J. He, C. A. Nowson, M. Lucas, G. A. MacGregor. "Increased consumption of fruit and vegetables is related to a reduced risk of coronary heart disease: meta-analysis of cohort studies." *Journal of Human Hypertension* 21 (2007): 717–28.

[101] F. J. He, C. A. Nowson, G. A. MacGregor. "Fruit and vegetable consumption and stroke: meta-analysis of cohort studies." *Lancet* 367 (2006): 320–26.

Dr. Mercola Non-GMO Shopping Guide: http://gmo.mercola.com/sites/gmo/shopping-guide.aspx

[102] P.K. Chelule, M.P. Mokoena, N. Gqaleni. "Advantages of traditional lactic acid bacteria fermentation of food in Africa." http://www.formatex.info/microbiology2/1160-1167.pdf

[103] G. Marks. *Encyclopedia of Jewish Food.* (Hoboken: Wiley, 2010).

[104] P.K. Chelule, M.P. Mokoena, N. Gqaleni. "Advantages of traditional lactic acid bacteria fermentation of food in Africa." http://www.formatex.info/microbiology2/1160-1167.pdf

[105] D. Paddon-Jones. "Protein, Weight Management, and Satiety." *American Journal of Clinical Nutrition* 87 (2008): 1558S–1561S.

[106] S. S. Yadav, et al. "USDA Nutrition Database: Lentils, Mature Seeds, Cooked, Boiled, Without Salt." Harvard School of Public Health (2007). http://www.hsph.harvard.edu/nutritionsource/protein/

[107] J. Pittaway, et al. "Effects of a Controlled Diet Supplemented with Chickpeas on Serum Lipids, Glucose Tolerance, Satiety and Bowel Function." *Journal of the American College of Nutrition* 26 (2007): 334–340.

M. Murty, J. Pittaway, M. J. Ball. "Chickpea Supplementation in an Australian Diet Affects Food Choice, Satiety and Bowel Health. Appetite." 54, no 2 (2010): 282–8.

"Iron." Office of Dietary Supplements (Accessed: 6/20/2013). http:// ods.od.nih.gov/factsheets/Iron-HealthProfessional.

"Folate." Office of Dietary Supplements; (Accessed: 6/20/2013). http:// ods.od.nih.gov/factsheets/Folate-HealthProfessional.

[108] Source: University of Illinois Extension

[109] C. J. Andersen, C. N. Blesso, J. Lee, J. Barona, D. Shah, M. J. Thomas, M. L. Fernandez. "Egg Consumption Modulates HDL Lipid Composition and Increases the Cholesterol-Accepting Capacity of Serum in Metabolic Syndrome." *Lipids* 48, no 6 (2013): 7–67.

K. L. Pearce, P. M. Clifton, M. Noakes. "Egg consumption as part of an energy-restricted high-protein diet improves blood glucose profiles in individuals with type 2 diabetes." *British Journal of Nutrition* 105, no 4 (2011): 584–92.

[110] N. Dhurandhar, J. Vander Wal, et al. "Egg breakfast enhances weight loss." *FASEB Journal* 21 (2007): 538.1.

[111] M. N. Ballesteros, R. M. Cabrera. "Dietary cholesterol does not increase biomarkers for chronic disease in a pediatric population from northern Mexico." *American Journal of Clinical Nutrition* 80, no. 4 (2004): 855–61.

[112] S. Samman, F. Kung, L. Carter, M. Foster, Z. Ahmad, J. Phuyal, P. Petocz. "Fatty acid composition of certified organic, conventional and Omega-3 eggs." *Food Chemistry* 116 (2009): 911–914.

[113] C. R. Sirtori. "Risks and benefits of soy phytoestrogens in cardiovascular diseases, cancer, climacteric symptoms and osteoporosis." *Drug Safety* 24, no. 9 (2001): 665–82.

[114] F. M. Sacks, A. Lichtenstein, L. Van Horn, W. Harris, P. Kris-Etherton, M. Winston— American Heart Association Nutrition Committee. "Soy protein, isoflavones, and cardiovascular health: an American Heart Association Science Advisory for professionals from the Nutrition Committee." *Circulation* 113, no. 7 (2006):1034–44.

[115] M. Messina, G. Redmond. "Effects of Soy Protein and Soybean Isoflavones on Thyroid Function in Healthy Adults and Hypothyroid Patients: A Review of the Relevant Literature." *Thyroid* 16, no. 3 (2006): 249–258.

E. Balk, M. Chung, P. Chew, et al. "Effects of Soy on Health Outcomes. Evidence Report/Technology Assessment no. 126." (Rockville, MD: Agency for Healthcare Research and Quality, 2005).

T. Low Dog. "Menopause: a review of botanical dietary supplements." *American Journal of Medicine* (suppl 12B) 118 (2005): 98S–108S.

F. M. Sacks, A. Lichtenstein, L. Van Horn, et al. "Soy protein, isoflavones, and cardiovascular health: an American Heart Association Science Advisory for professionals from the Nutrition Committee." *Circulation*. 113, no. 7 (2006): 1034–1044.

"Soy." Natural Medicines Comprehensive Database Web site. (Accessed: 07/23/2009). http://www.naturaldatabase.com.

"Soy (Glycine max [L.] Merr.)." Natural Standard Database Web site. (Accessed: 07/23/2009). http://www.naturalstandard.com.

"Non-GMO Shopping Guide." Mercola.com. http://mercola.fileburst.com/PDF/GMObrochure.pdf

[116] C. Bennet. "15 Tips to Breeze Through the Holidays Without Overeating." HuffingtonPost.com. (Accessed: 06/20/13). http://www.huffingtonpost.com/connie-bennett/thanksgiving-15-tips-to-b_b_787057.html.

[117] K. van Ittersum, B. Wansink. "Plate Size and Color Suggestibility: The Delboeuf Illusion's Bias on Serving and Eating Behavior." *Journal of Consumer Research* (2012).

[118] T. Parker-Pope. "Unlocking the Benefits of Garlic." *The New York Times* (2007). http://well.blogs.nytimes.com/2007/10/15/unlocking-the-benefits-of-garlic/

[119] R. Hirano R, W. Sasamoto, A. Matsumoto, et al. "Antioxidant ability of various flavonoids against DPPH radicals and LDL oxidation." *Journal of Nutritional Science and Vitaminology* 47, no. 5 (2001): 357–62.

[120] A. Sengupta, S. Ghosh, S. Bhattacharjee. "Allium vegetables in cancer prevention: an overview." *Asian Pac J Cancer Prev* 5, no. 3 (2004): 237–45.

[121] V. A. Parthasarathy, B. Chempakam, T. Zachariah. *Chemistry of Spices* (Oxfordshire: Cabi, 2008).

[122] G. Cappello, M. Spezzaferro, L. Grossi, L. Manzoli, L. Marzio. "Peppermint oil (Mintoil) in the treatment of irritable bowel syndrome: a prospective double blind placebo-controlled randomized trial." *Digestive and Liver Disease* 39, no. 6 (2007): 530–6.

[123] D. L. McKay, J. B. Blumberg. "A review of the bioactivity and potential health benefits of peppermint tea (*Mentha piperita L.*)." *Phytotherapy Research* 20, no. 8 (2006): 619–33.

[124] M. Valussi. "Functional foods with digestion-enhancing properties." *International Journal of Food Sciences and Nutrition* (2011): 1–8.

ACKNOWLEDGMENTS

There are many people I have to thank for getting me to where I am, both in my personal and professional life.

A big thank you to all my patients for teaching me more than any textbook could. I am honored that you feel comfortable enough to let me into your lives and trust me to help. The goals you strive to accomplish, aside from whatever trials and tribulations you face, inspire me, and I am proud to be your dietitian.

A lot of what I aim to accomplish in my career could not be without the help of many professionals I look toward as mentors. A special thanks to Keri Gans, MS, RD, CDN, whose quick responses and generous advice helped me reach career goals I did not know I could. My staff is a super crew—thanks for all your help pulling the book together. Especially my assistant, Sarah Sarway.

To my agent, Jody Klein, Brandt and Hochman Literary Agents, Inc: You surpassed the preconception I had of a literary agent's role. Thank you for representing and supporting me with your detailed edits and being my "go-to" help for any questions, no matter how simple they were. I could not have written this book without your help.

A huge thank you to Skyhorse Publishing, for taking a chance on a first-time author, especially Nicole Frail, for sharing my enthusiasm for this book and helping to get my message out to the masses. A special thank you to my community and friends for their support.

My food photo shoot was truly a group effort with the help of Jessica Mathews from kosherfoodies.com, Stefanie Sakkal, whose contributions are too much to list, the Tawil's for graciously handing over the keys to their kitchen, Kitchen Caboodles for sharing sample props, and, of course, the talented Hannah Kaminsky, food stylist, and Meir Pliskin, photographer. Thank you to Lenore Cohen for her creative graphic design work. Thanks to Susie Kampf, Pink by Susie, for her fabulous makeup for the photo shoot.

None of what I do could happen without the support of my entire family: brothers, sisters, cousins, aunts, uncles, and grandparents—especially my mother-in-law, Rebecca, for running over to help with my children and sharing and cooking her recipes, and my mom, Aileen, for raising me with real-food recipes and home-cooked meals I could look forward to every day of my childhood. A special thank you to my brother, Abie, and brother-in-laws, Donny and Avi, for their input on Jewish law and biblical references.

To my wonderful children, who show me what it means to enjoy life and be happy every day. I owe a huge thank you for bearing with me when Mommy had to spend time writing and working. Everything I do is for you. And of course, my husband, Elliot. Thank you for taking on more than your share of Daddy duties and supporting me throughout the writing process. I love you all so much!

"And you will eat, and you will be satisfied, and you will bless the Lord your God" (Deut. 8:10).

Most importantly, thank you to G–d for allowing my dreams of writing a book to become a reality, and for the opportunity to help better the lives of those who read it. May we all be blessed to recognize all of the ways G–d's loving presence supports and sustains us, even in the most routine aspects of our lives.

INDEX

Index

and trans fat on Nutrition Facts panels, 55
fennel, 235, 290–291
Fennel Soup, 290–291
fermented grains, 98
fermented soy, 153–154
fermented vegetables (pickling), 128–130, 222–225
fiber. *see also* whole grains
    and carbohydrates, 102,
      111–112, 187
    in chia seeds, 73
    dietary, and weight management (chart), 103
    Dietary Guidelines for Americans (2005), 104
    and food labels, reading,
      186, 187
    fortification process versus real foods, 103,
      187
    high fiber diets, benefits of, 111, 119, 121
    insoluble fiber, 102, 119, 137
    intake, and "stop eating" signals acquired
      from, 28–29
    in legumes, 137, 138
    in nuts, 188
    soluble fiber, 137
    sources of (fruits/vegetables), 29, 31, 102, 117
fish
    anchovies and sardines, 149–150
    kosher, and Omega-3 content, 146–147
    kosher diet, 16
    Recipes
      Lemony, Lemon of
        Sole, 267
      Mini Fish Sticks with Homemade Tartar
        Dipping Sauce, 276
      Moroccan Fish, 286–288
      Pesto Crusted
        Salmon, 265
      Salmon Burger, 274
      Salmon Za'atar
        Skewers, 270
    shopping list for kosher real foods, 202
    wild versus farmed,
      148–149, 202
flavonoids, 71, 117–118
flaxseeds, 72–73, 75, 145
fluid intake and hydration.
    see also beverages
    alcohol, 39
    coffee, 38–39
    water requirements, 36–38
folic acid (folate), 91, 117,
    120, 137
Food & Function journal, 71
food allergies
    common, 156
    cow's milk, 83–84, 89
    and eating out, 166

and kosher symbols, 193
and non-dairy alternative milk sources, 89, 92
soy foods, 156
Food and Drug Administration (FDA). *see* FDA
    (Food and Drug Administration)
food industry. *see also* supermarkets
    100-calorie snack packs, misleading health
      marketing, 46–47, 188
    actual versus perceived healthiness of food
      and, 2–4
    GMOs, and labeling not required for in US,
      127
    lack of trust IN for real-food choices, 86
    low-fat and fat-free craze, and health
      misconceptions regarding, 48–50
    misleading terms, 144
    organic, and perception of healthiness, 3, 122,
      123–124, 191–192
    processed foods, and brain chemistry changes,
      47–48, 304nn18–20
    real versus perceived healthiness and, 19
    trans fats, and food labelling misconceptions,
      55
Food Journals (Food and Mood Diary), 31–33, 34,
    38, 40,
    85, 111
free-range eggs. *see* eggs
freezer items, shopping list for, 204–205
fruit. *see* vegetables/fruits

garbanzo beans. *see* chickpeas (garbanzo beans)
garlic, 218
Garlicky String Beans, 245
gelatin, 16
genistein, 151
ghrelin, 35–36
GI (glycemic index). *see* glycemic index (GI)
gluconeogenesis, 24
gluten intolerance, 96–97, 105, 112–114
gluten-free trend, 96
glycemic index (GI), 9, 26,
    29–30, 99, 102, 108
GMOs (genetically modified organisms), 127–128,
    155, 198
goat's milk, 89–90
goitrogens, 155, 157
grains. *see* whole grains
Guide to the Perplexed, 3:48 (Moses Maimonides),
    18–19

Hamid (A Twist on Vegetable Soup), 289
Harvard School of Public Health, 26, 54, 82, 117,
    152
Healthier Mac 'N' Cheese, 257
Healthy Apple Crisp, 298–299
heart disease, 58, 117, 120, 142

Index

Index

Index